PRIMER *of*

Arthroscopy

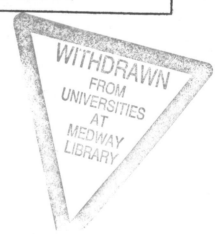

PRIMER *of*

Arthroscopy

Mark D. Miller, MD

S. Ward Casscells Professor of Orthopaedics
Head, Division of Sports Medicine
University of Virginia
Charlottesville, Virginia;
Team Physician, James Madison University,
Harrisonburg, Virginia

A. Bobby Chhabra, MD

Vice-Chairman, Orthopaedic Surgery
Charles J. Frankel Professor of Orthopaedic
    Surgery
Professor of Plastic Surgery
Division Head, Hand and Upper Extremity
    Surgery
Director, UVA Hand Center
University of Virginia Health System
Charlottesville, Virginia

Marc R. Safran, MD

Professor, Orthopaedic Surgery
Associate Director, Sports Medicine
Fellowship Director, Sports Medicine
Team Physician
Stanford University
Redwood City, California

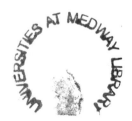

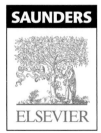
SAUNDERS

ELSEVIER

SAUNDERS
ELSEVIER

1600 John F. Kennedy Blvd.
Ste 1800
Philadelphia, PA 19103-2899

PRIMER OF ARTHROSCOPY   ISBN: 978-1-4377-0155-5

Notice

Knowledge and best practice in this field are constantly changing. As new research and experience broaden our knowledge, changes in practice, treatment and drug therapy may become necessary or appropriate. Readers are advised to check the most current information provided (i) on procedures featured or (ii) by the manufacturer of each product to be administered, to verify the recommended dose or formula, the method and duration of administration, and contraindications. It is the responsibility of the practitioner, relying on their own experience and knowledge of the patient, to make diagnoses, to determine dosages and the best treatment for each individual patient, and to take all appropriate safety precautions. To the fullest extent of the law, neither the Publisher nor the Editors assumes any liability for any injury and/or damage to persons or property arising out of or related to any use of the material contained in this book.

The Publisher

Library of Congress Cataloging-in-Publication Data
Miller, Mark D.
  Primer of arthroscopy / Mark D. Miller, A. Bobby Chhabra, Marc R. Safran. — 1st ed.
      p. ; cm.
  Includes bibliographical references.
  ISBN 978-1-4377-0155-5
  1. Joints—Endoscopic surgery. 2. Arthroscopy. I. Chhabra, Anikar. II. Safran, Marc R. III. Title.
      [DNLM: 1. Arthroscopy—methods—Handbooks. 2. Arthroscopy—adverse effects—Handbooks. WE 39 M6495p 2010]
  RD686.M55 2010
  617.4'720597—dc22

                                                            2010012491

Publishing Director: Kimberly Murphy
Developmental Editor: Agnes H. Byrne
Publishing Services Manager: Hemamalini Rajendrababu
Project Manager: Srikumar Narayanan
Designer: Steven Stave

Working together to grow
libraries in developing countries

www.elsevier.com | www.bookaid.org | www.sabre.org

ELSEVIER   BOOK AID International   Sabre Foundation

Printed in the United States of America

Last digit is the print number: 9 8 7 6 5 4 3 2 1

Foreword

Dr. Robert W. Jackson was asked by Dr. Mark D. Miller to write the Foreword for PRIMER OF ARTHROSCOPY, and he agreed. Unfortunately Bob Jackson, a Canadian pioneer in the field of arthroscopy and sports medicine, passed away after a battle with pancreatic cancer before he could honor Mark's request. Mark asked if I would contribute the Foreword, and I am honored and humbled to pick up the torch for my mentor, Bob Jackson. Bob was a kind man, a true leader, and a surgeon among surgeons. It was back in 1984 when I went to Toronto that Bob taught me about arthroscopy.

Bob was always very complimentary and thoroughly impressed with Mark's work and that of his co-editors, Drs. Marc R. Safran and A. Bobby Chhabra. Mark Miller was my sports medicine fellow here at Pitt in 1993, as was Marc Safran one year later. I worked with them here in Pittsburgh, and now they are leaders in the field and teaching arthroscopy to their fellows. They, in turn, are training the next generation of fellows. All of us arthroscopists stand on the shoulder of giants–giants like Bob Jackson.

Bob introduced the technique of arthroscopy to the western world in 1965, and it entirely revolutionized sports medicine. Over the course of his distinguished career he received many awards too numerous to list. In 1994 *Sports Illustrated* named him one of the 40 individuals who changed the games we play and watch with the introduction of arthroscopic surgery. In addition to his extraordinary surgical skills Bob was admired by all for his kindness, integrity, and humility.

In PRIMER OF ARTHROSCOPY Dr. Mark Miller and his co-authors will present to residents and beginning arthroscopists the technique introduced by Bob Jackson.

Freddie H. Fu, MD, DSc (Hon), DPs (Hon)
David Silver Professor and Chairman
Department of Orthopaedic Surgery
University of Pittsburgh School of Medicine
Distinguished Service Professor
Head Team Physician
University of Pittsburgh
Athletic Department Past Present
American Orthopaedic Society for Sports Medicine
President, International Society of Arthroscopy, Knee Surgery, and Orthopedic Sports Medicine

PREFACE

Although there are a plethora of Arthroscopy textbooks out there, including some that we have contributed to and/or edited, there is nothing available for the beginning arthroscopist. Teaching the art and science of arthroscopy to the novice is one of the most challenging things that we do in postgraduate education. Sometimes it is rewarding, but often it is frustrating . . . for both the teacher and the student! Therefore, we set out to create this text . . . it is what it is – a *Primer of Arthroscopy*. The word "primer," as defined by Dictionary.com (and where else should you go for this generation of students) is defined as "an elementary book for teaching children to read." We purposely have made this book elementary – basic training in arthroscopy. We all have often compared resident education to teaching our children, so that is appropriate. And, although we are not teaching our "kids" to read, we are trying to teach them to arthroscopically operate in a skillful, safe, and efficient fashion.

We have organized this text anatomically, beginning with the knee. We chose to begin with the knee because that is the most commonly performed arthroscopy, and it is where most surgeons begin to use the scope. This is true from an historical perspective and from a training perspective. Hip and ankle arthroscopy follow. The shoulder is the most common upper extremity joint for arthroscopy, and so this is chapter has been given special emphasis. The elbow and wrist chapters complete the upper extremity and round out the text. Each chapter is organized just as one should approach each case. Following a brief introduction, preoperative considerations are discussed. This is followed by a review of examination under anesthesia and positioning. A detailed description of anatomy precedes a description of portal placement and diagnostic arthroscopy, because it forms the basis for a thorough understanding of that joint. Each chapter concludes with an overview of common procedures and a discussion of complications, and how to avoid them. The text has been created in a bulleted easy-to-read format and is replete with clear color illustrations. One of the highlights of the book is the enclosed DVD with a collection of narrated arthroscopy videos, both original and from the Elsevier library.

We would like to thank the staff of Elsevier for their help in putting together this *Primer*. Between the three of us, we have had the privilege to educate hundreds of residents and fellows of varying abilities directly; and thousands of others, nationally and internationally, indirectly. We hope this book makes it easier to master the skills of diagnostic and operative arthroscopy, and lead a new generation of arthroscopists into the future.

Mark D. Miller
A. Bobby Chhabra
Marc R. Safran

CONTRIBUTORS

A. Bobby Chhabra, MD
Vice-Chairman, Orthopaedic Surgery
Charles J. Frankel Professor of Orthopaedic Surgery
Professor of Plastic Surgery
Division Head, Hand and Upper Extremity Surgery
Director, UVA Hand Center
University of Virginia Health System
Charlottesville, Virginia

Sanaz Hariri, MD
Fellow, Sports Medicine
Stanford University
Redwood City, California

Jennifer A. Hart, MPAS, PA-C
Physician Assistant
University of Virginia
Department of Orthopaedic Surgery
Division of Sports Medicine
Charlottesville, Virginia

Kenneth J. Hunt, MD
Assistant Professor
Orthopaedic Surgery
Stanford University
Redwood City, California

Mark D. Miller, MD
S. Ward Casscells Professor of Orthopaedics
Head, Division of Sports Medicine
University of Virginia
Charlottesville, Virginia;
Team Physician, James Madison University,
Harrisonburg, Virginia

Sara D. Rynders, MPAS, PA-C
Physician Assistant
UVA Hand Center
Department of Orthopaedic Surgery
Division of Hand & Upper Extremity Surgery
University of Virginia Health System
Charlottesville, Virginia

Marc R. Safran, MD
Professor, Orthopaedic Surgery
Associate Director, Sports Medicine
Fellowship Director, Sports Medicine
Team Physician
Stanford University
Redwood City, California

Zackary D. Vaughn, MD
Fellow, Sports Medicine
Stanford University
Redwood City, California

Melissa D. Willenborg, MD
Resident
Department of Orthopaedic Surgery
University of Virginia
Charlottesville, Virginia

TABLE OF CONTENTS

CHAPTER 1

OVERVIEW OF ARTHROSCOPY

Mark D. Miller

History of Arthroscopy

- The use of an endoscopic device for internal examination dates back to the early 1800s but it wasn't until a century later that the first documented knee joint examination was performed.

- The clinical use of arthroscopy, originally referred to as "arthro-endoscopy," is generally thought to have been simultaneously developed by Dr. Eugen Bircher of Switzerland and a Japanese professor named Kenji Takagi.

- The first paper in the United States on the topic of arthroscopy was published by Dr. Phillip Kreuscher on the diagnosis and treatment of meniscal tears.

- In the 1930s, Dr. Michael Burman from the Hospital for Joint Diseases in New York published the first arthroscopic images in his paper "Arthroscopy or the Direct Visualization of Joints."

- World War II slowed progress in the field for the next few decades but after the war Dr. Masake Watanabe took over previous work and introduced the first fiberoptic arthroscope, introduced the concept of triangulation using various portals, and performed the first arthroscopic meniscectomy.

- Largely due to his efforts in teaching, he was later elected the first chairman of the International Arthroscopy Association (IAA) when it was founded in 1972.

- Robert W. Jackson, a Canadian surgeon who visited Dr. Watanabe, brought interest and experience back to other surgeons in North America. He gave the first instructional course lecture on arthroscopy at the American Academy of Orthopaedic Surgeons in 1968.

- Dr. Richard O'Connor also visited Dr. Watanabe and pioneered some of the early advances in indications and techniques for arthroscopy.

- Ward Casscells and Jack McGinty were among the early North American advocates for arthroscopy who continued to develop this surgical field after spending time with Dr. Jackson.

- These men were among the founders of the Arthroscopy Association of North American (AANA) which was established in 1981 as a subgroup of the IAA. Its primary goal was and still is "to promote, encourage, support and foster through continuing medical education functions, the development and dissemination of knowledge in the discipline of arthroscopic surgery."

Arthroscopic Equipment

- Arthroscope
  - Fiberoptic instrument which is introduced into a joint via a cannula.
  - A fiberoptic cable and camera attached to the arthroscope allow visualization of the interior joint structures.
  - Arthroscopes are classified by their diameter and viewing angle.
  - View is magnified.
  - Variable amount is based on distance to object being viewed.
  - It is best to compare against a known reference.
  - Lens is angled *(Fig. 1-1)*.
  - View is typically opposite the light cord.
  - 30-degree lens is used most often.
  - 70-degree lens can be helpful to look "around corners."
  - Different sizes are available.
  - 4 mm is used for larger joints (knee and shoulder).
  - 2.5 mm is used for intermediate joints (ankle).
  - 1.9 mm is used for smaller joints (wrist).

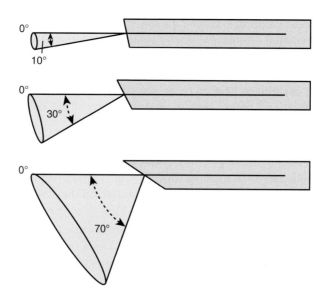

Figure 1-1. The angled lens of the arthroscope.

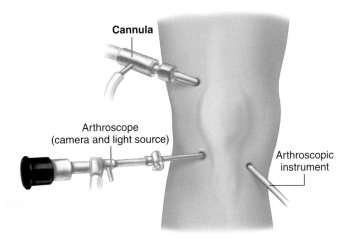

Figure 1-2. The arthroscopic cannula.

- Cannulas *(Fig. 1-2)*
  - Arthroscopic cannula allows fluid ingress/egress and arthroscope locks into it.
  - Typically, they are introduced with a blunt trocar to minimize iatrogenic injury.
  - Disposable cannulas can be used in established portals.
- Camera
  - Becoming increasingly precise
  - Number of "chips" related to resolution of image
- Light Source
  - Allows maximum lumens
  - Connected via fiberoptic cord
- Monitor *(Fig. 1-3)*
  - Television
  - Resolution continues to improve.
  - Monitor should be placed on the top of the tower to allow the best visualization from the surgical field.
- Image Capture System *(Fig. 1-4)*
  - Digital and video images can be captured and stored electronically.
  - They can be stored and edited for clinical and educational purposes.

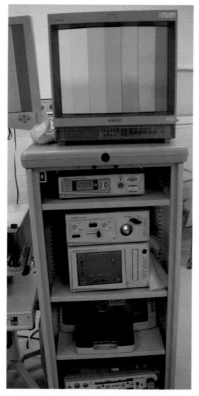

Figure 1-3. The arthroscopic monitor sits on top of the tower to allow easy visual access by the surgeon.

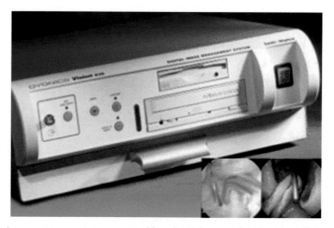

Figure 1-4. Image capture systems can provide printed images, digital copies of images, or even videography as selected by the surgeon. *(From St. Pierre P. Instrumentation and equipment. In Miller MD, Cole BJ. Textbook of Arthroscopy, Philadelphia, Elsevier, 2004, p 13.)*

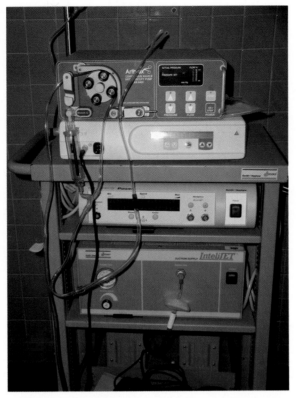

Figure 1-5. Fluid management may be obtained by gravity-based or pump-based systems. *(From St. Pierre P. Instrumentation and equipment. In Miller MD, Cole BJ. Textbook of Arthroscopy, Philadelphia, Elsevier, 2004, p 10.)*

- Editing and archiving requires constant attention.

- Software and options continue to improve.

- **Fluid Management System** *(Fig. 1-5)*
  - Irrigation is necessary during arthroscopy to distend the joint, improve visualization, and remove debris.

  - Gravity devices have been largely supplanted by computer-driven pumps.

  - Pumps can allow for constant pressure in the joint and can be increased if bleeding develops to obtain hemostasis.

  - The use of epinephrine in the fluid can help reduce bleeding.

- **Hand-held Instruments** *(Fig. 1-6)*
  - Probe is basic instrument that allows a sense of touch.

  - Include baskets (also known as biters or punches), grabbers, and scissors, all of which allow trimming of joint structures.

  - Different angles and shapes enhance placement in the joint.

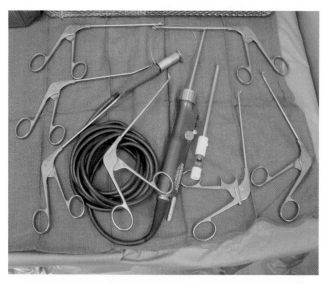

Figure 1-6. A variety of specialized hand-held instruments are manufactured for arthroscopic use including baskets, graspers, probes, and shavers.

- Motorized Shavers
    - Allow removal of unwanted material in the joint
    - Disposable and available in a variety of sizes and shapes *(Fig. 1-7)*
    - "Aggressiveness" of blades should be determined based on task at hand.

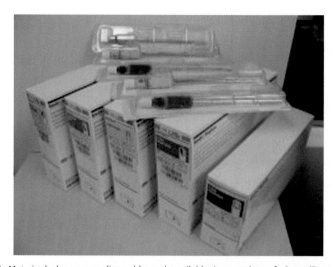

Figure 1-7. Motorized shavers are disposable and available in a variety of sizes. *(From St. Pierre P. Instrumentation and equipment. In Miller MD, Cole BJ. Textbook of Arthroscopy, Philadelphia, Elsevier, 2004, p 11.)*

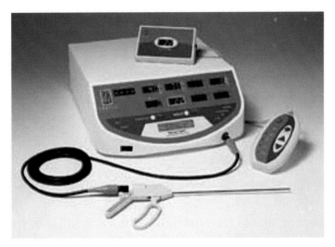

Figure 1-8. An example of a thermal device for delivering radiofrequency energy. *(From St. Pierre P. Instrumentation and equipment. In Miller MD, Cole BJ. Textbook of Arthroscopy, Philadelphia, Elsevier, 2004, p 13.)*

- Thermal Devices *(Fig. 1-8)*
  - "Shrinkage" type devices have largely fallen out of favor.
  - Ablative devices that use radiofrequency (RF) energy are popular for procedures such as notchplasty (knee) and acromioplasty (shoulder).
- Specialty Instruments *(Fig. 1-9)*
  - Procedure-specific
  - Guides for tunnel placement, implant delivering devices, fixation devices, suture passage, and a variety of other instruments are available.
  - It is important to be apprised of current developments.

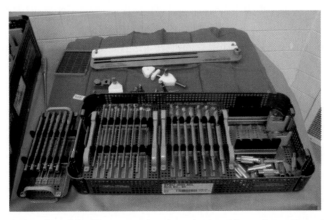

Figure 1-9. A variety of specialized instruments have been developed for use in specific surgical techniques.

Arthroscopic Team and Support

- Surgeon
  - Captain of the ship
  - The surgeon is ultimately responsible for all aspects of the patient's operative experience.
- Assistant
  - Assists with visualization and instrumentation
  - This may be another surgeon, resident, physician assistant, or scrub nurse.
  - The assistant should have adequate understanding of sterile technique and use of arthroscopic equipment.
- Scrub Nurse
  - This person is responsible for assisting the surgeon with the equipment.
  - For maximum efficiency, the scrub nurse should be trained and experienced in the use of arthroscopic and special arthroscopic instruments.
- Circulating Nurse
  - The circulating nurse is an important liaison between the other members of the surgical team.
  - Knowledge of the setup of the arthroscopic equipment is important.
- Surgery Center
  - Should have operative suites of an adequate size to house the somewhat bulky arthroscopic tower and equipment while still allowing room for the staff to move safely around the sterile field
  - Should allow for storage facilities for the variety of special arthroscopic equipment within easy access to the surgical suite
  - Should have sufficient and knowledgeable staff to allow for efficient turnover and successful teamwork
  - OSHA guidelines must be followed.
- Equipment Acquisition
  - Balancing equipment costs versus emerging technology is a constant battle but functioning up-to-date equipment is important to keep up with advancement in technique.

- Equipment Maintenance and Sterilization
  - Equipment must be maintained including careful periodic examination for broken or loose pieces.

  - The arthroscope and its cables cannot be treated with standard autoclaving.

  - Gas sterilization using ethylene oxide is effective but requires excessively long turnover times, making this method inadequate for busy surgical practices.

  - High-level disinfection systems such as those using peracetic acid (Steris, Menor, Ohio) have largely replaced true sterilization.

Arthroscopic Basics

- Rotating the arthroscope allows the surgeon to see in different directions.
  - A 30-degree arthroscope can give you a 60-degree field of view *(Fig. 1-10)*
- Keep a perspective.
  - Get a "press box" view.

  - Remember that objects viewed through the arthroscope are magnified and the degree is dependent on the distance of the lens from the object.

  - Use an instrument of a known size to help estimate the size of the object being observed.

- Have a "home base"
  - When in doubt, reorient yourself back to a known anatomic location.

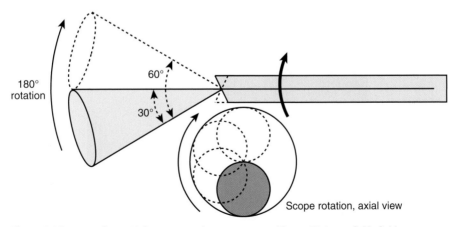

Figure 1-10. By rotating a 30-degree scope, the surgeon can achieve a 60-degree field of vision.

- In the knee, use the notch.
- In the shoulder, use the biceps anchor.
- **Never injure normal structures.**
  - Do not force instruments into the joint.
  - See where your instruments are and protect where they should not be.
- **Keep your "wings level."**
  - The camera cord of the arthroscope should always face toward the foot.
- **Keep the area of interest in the middle of the visual field.**
- **Keep the overall anatomy of the joint in mind.**
  - Move either the arthroscope or the instrument, not both.
- **Hold the scope in one hand and the instrument in the opposite hand.**
- **Triangulate.**
- **Depth perception is a matter of experience.**
- **Shaver Rules** *(Fig. 1-11)*
  - See the shaver.
  - See what you are shaving.
  - See what you are protecting.
  - Do not shave the end of the arthroscope!

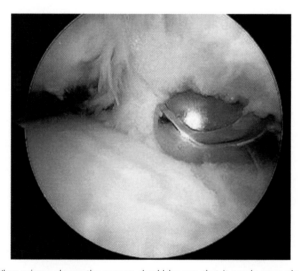

Figure 1-11. When using a shaver, the surgeon should be sure that it can be seen along with the area being shaved, and any area being protected.

- Rub or brush the material you are shaving. Direct contact yields the best results.

- Control the suction: Bubbles = too much suction; Floaters = too little suction.

REFERENCES

Baer GS and Sekiya JK. Knee arthroscopy—the basics. In Miller MD, Cole BJ, Cosgarea AJ, and Sekiya JK (eds). *Sports Knee Surgery*, Philadelphia, Elsevier, 2008; pp 23–39.

Ishibashi Y and Yamamoto Y. The History of Arthroscopy. In Miller MD and Cole BJ (eds). *Textbook of Arthroscopy*, Philadelphia, Elsevier, 2004.

Jackson RW. History of Arthroscopy. In McGinty JB and Jackson RW (eds). *Operative Arthroscopy*, 2nd ed. Philadelphia, Lippincott, 1996.

Miller MD, Cole BJ, Cosgarea AJ, and Sekiya JK. *Sports Knee Surgery*, Philadelphia, Elsevier, 2008.

Miller MD, Howard RF, and Plancher KD. *Surgical Atlas of Sports Medicine*, Philadelphia, Elsevier, 2003.

Miller MD and Sekiya JK. Knee Arthroscopy. In Miller MD and Sekiya JK (eds). *Core Knowledge in Orthopaedics: Sports Medicine*, Philadelphia, Elsevier, 2006, pp 22–26.

Ong BC, Shen FH, Musahl V, Fu FH, and Diduch DR. Knee: Patient positioning, portal placement, and normal arthroscopy anatomy. In Miller MD and Cole BJ (eds). *Textbook of Arthroscopy*; Philadelphia, Elsevier, 2004; pp 463–469.

KNEE ARTHROSCOPY

Mark D. Miller and Jennifer A. Hart

Introduction

- The knee was the first joint to be examined arthroscopically and many of the fundamental principles for arthroscopy were originally developed for the knee.
  - First knee arthroscopy was performed in Europe.
  - Japanese surgeons (Takagi and Watanabe) significantly advanced the field.
  - North American surgeons did not embrace knee arthroscopy until the 1960s (Jackson, O'Connor, Casscells, McGinty)
- Knee arthroscopy quickly progressed from a diagnostic to a therapeutic modality.
- Like any joint, a systematic evaluation of the entire knee should precede treatment. Documentation, including images of all pathology and treatment thereof, should be kept in the patient's medical records.
- Indications
  - Synovitis
  - Meniscal tear
  - Septic knee joint
  - Anterior cruciate ligament tear
  - Mild-to-moderate knee arthritis with mechanical symptoms.
  - Focal chondral defect
  - Loose bodies
  - Failure of conservative treatment with continued knee pain that affects patient activity.
- Common procedures performed include
  - Diagnostic arthroscopy
  - Synovectomy
  - Loose body removal
  - Partial meniscectomy
  - Meniscus repair

- Loose body removal
- Chondroplasty
- Microfracture
- Osteochondral plug transfer
- Autologous chondrocyte implantation
- Anterior cruciate ligament reconstruction

- Contraindications to knee arthroscopy include
  - Local skin infection over portal site
  - Patients who are expected to be noncompliant with postoperative rehabilitation

Preoperative Considerations

- A thorough medical evaluation, to include a complete history and physical examination and review of symptoms, should be reviewed before performing arthroscopy.
  - Preoperative consultation with appropriate primary care/medical specialists and anesthesia will help reduce perioperative problems.
  - Postoperative deep vein thrombosis (DVT) prophylaxis should be considered for patients with several risk factors (smokers, older patients, females on birth control pills, patients with known history of DVT, obese patients, etc.)
- Review all medical records and *sign your site!*
- Anesthetic options include local, regional, and general anesthesia, or some combination thereof.
  - Local anesthesia alone is best suited for short, simple procedures such as loose body removal. More extensive procedures and stressing the knee to evaluate compartments are poorly tolerated.
  - Regional anesthesia including spinal, epidural and selective nerve blocks can be useful alone or in combination with general anesthesia for prolonged postoperative pain relief (e.g., outpatient anterior cruciate ligament [ACL] surgery).
  - General anesthesia is favored for the majority of patients. It allows for complete exposure, muscle relaxation, and obviates any problems with tourniquet pain.
- Examination under anesthesia (EUA)
  - Best performed before placing the leg into a leg holder
  - Systematic physical examination should be performed.

- Positioning *(Fig. 2-1)*
  - The patient is placed supine. A commercially available leg holder or post is used to stabilize the thigh during examination under anesthesia.
  - Nonoperative leg should be padded and protected.
  - Standard prep and drape is accomplished.
- Equipment
  - Arthroscope
    - 30-degree scope most commonly used but 70-degree scope can be helpful for areas that may be otherwise difficult to see (e.g., posterior corners).
  - Arthroscopic probe
    - Allows the surgeon the "sense of touch"
  - Hand-held instruments
    - Up-going instruments best for medial compartment
    - Straight instruments more useful in lateral compartment
    - Right and left angled instruments often helpful in contouring menisci.
  - Motorized instruments
    - Helpful for removing debris and contouring
    - Larger (5.5 mm) shavers best for synovium/central areas
    - Smaller (4.5 mm) shavers best in the compartments (avoid chondral injury)

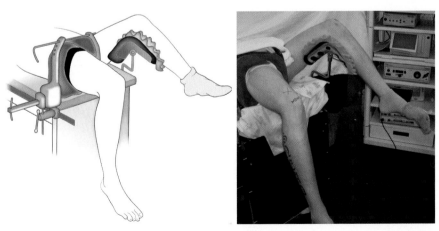

Figure 2-1. The patient is positioned supine with the use of a leg holder or lateral post. *(From Miller MD, Chhabra AB, Hurwitz S, et al. [eds]. Orthopaedic Surgical Approaches. Philadelphia, Elsevier, 2008, p 483.)*

Relevant Anatomy *(Fig. 2-2)*

- Patella
  - Thickest articular cartilage
  - Articulates with the femoral trochlea
    - ▸ Fully engages at 30- to 40-degrees of knee flexion
- Distal Femur
  - Sulcus terminalis lateral
  - Medial condyle is larger than the lateral condyle.
  - Lateral condyle is longer but narrower.
- Proximal Tibia
  - Cruciates central
    - ▸ Insert between tibial spines.
    - ▸ The ACL is more anterior and inserts on the lateral femoral condyle.
    - ▸ The posterior cruciate ligament (PCL) originates posteriorly, below the articular surface, and inserts on the medial femoral condyle.

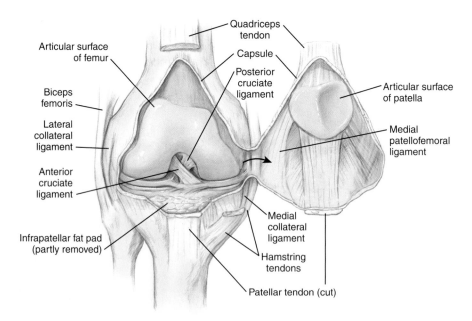

Figure 2-2. The anatomy of the knee joint. *(From Miller MD, Chhabra AB, Hurwitz S, et al. [eds]. Orthopaedic Surgical Approaches. Philadelphia, Elsevier, 2008, p 428.)*

▸ Medial tibial plateau is longer in sagittal plane and is concave.

▸ Lateral tibial plateau is convex in the sagittal plane.

▸ Menisci cover the tibial plateaus.

■ Medial meniscus is more "C-shaped" and insertions are far apart.

■ Lateral meniscus is more semicircular and insertions are adjacent to the ACL.

Portal Placement *(Fig. 2-3)*

● Inferolateral portal

■ Just lateral to patellar tendon and just above the joint line

■ Primary viewing portal

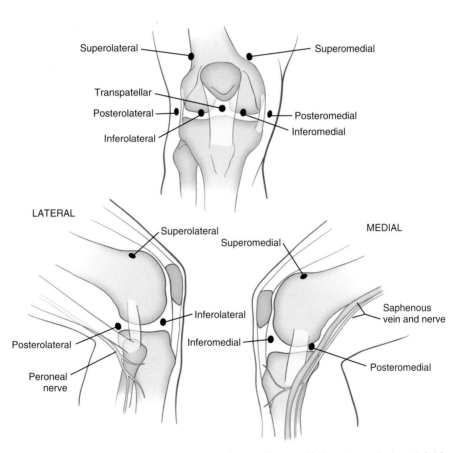

Figure 2-3. Portal placement for knee arthroscopy. *(From Miller MD, Chhabra AB, Hurwitz S, et al. [eds]. Orthopaedic Surgical Approaches. Philadelphia, Elsevier, 2008, p 485.)*

- Inferomedial portal
  - Just medial to the patellar tendon and just above the joint line
  - Usually easier to palpate and lateral portal location can be based on this portal.
  - Primary instrument portal
  - Can be used for visualization based on access
- Superior portals
  - Created above the level of the patella
  - Lateral favored (does not disrupt the vastus medialis obliquus)
  - Can be used to observe patellar tracking
- Posteromedial portal
  - Just posterior to the medial collateral ligament (MCL), above the joint line
  - Localized with spinal needle
  - Avoid saphenous nerve/vein (nick and spread)
  - Used for viewing posterior horn medial meniscus, loose body removal, complete synovectomy
- Posterolateral portal
  - Just posterior to the lateral collateral ligament (LCL) but anterior to biceps, above joint line
  - Localized with spinal needle
  - Avoid peroneal nerve (posterior to biceps)
  - Used for viewing posterior horn of lateral meniscus, loose body removal, complete synovectomy.
- Additional portals (e.g., posterior portals)
  - As needed
  - Useful for extensive synovectomies

Diagnostic Arthroscopy *(Fig. 2-4)*

- Scope insertion
  - The anterolateral portal is made with an 11-blade (sharp edge superior) and the capsule is incised by aiming toward the femoral notch.
  - The scope cannula with blunt obturator is inserted into the inferolateral portal and directed up into the suprapatellar pouch by extending the knee and "bouncing" off the medial femoral condyle—do not force the obturator!

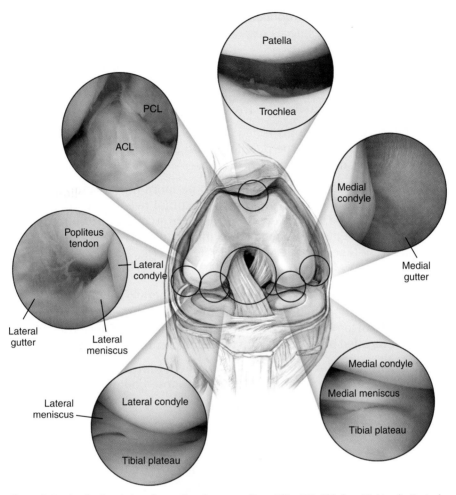

Figure 2-4. Visualization during diagnostic arthroscopy. *(From Miller MD, Chhabra AB, Hurwitz S, et al. [eds]. Orthopaedic Surgical Approaches. Philadelphia, Elsevier, 2008, p 486.)*

- ■ The final position can be confirmed by sweeping the obturator back and forth.

- ■ The anteromedial portal can be made at the outset of the case, or it can be localized under direct visualization with a spinal needle.

- ■ The obturator is removed and the scope is inserted into the cannula.

- ■ The scope is held with the camera cord down, facing the foot and the light cord is rotated to change the direction of viewing.

- ● Suprapatellar pouch
  - ■ The suprapatellar pouch is visualized both medially and laterally, looking for synovitis, loose bodies, plicae, or adhesions.

- A shaver can be introduced through the inferomedial or a superior portal as necessary.

- Patellofemoral joint
  - The arthroscope is withdrawn and the undersurface of the patella can be visualized. The lens is rotated and the entire surface of the patella is characterized.

  - The trochlea is also inspected and the articulation with the patella is assessed. The patella should be fully engaged in the trochlea at about 40-degree flexion.

  - The patellofemoral articulation can be more fully visualized by using a far superior lateral portal. A spinal needle is used to localize the portal position and the arthroscope is introduced through the portal. Patellar tracking is studied as the knee is passively taken from extension to flexion (*Fig. 2-5*).

- Lateral gutter
  - The scope is taken over the lateral femoral condyle with the knee in extension. The scope is "lifted up" or retracted slightly to avoid scuffing the lateral femoral condyle. The scope must also be retracted slightly to be directed below a constant reflection of capsule in the gutter.

  - The entire gutter (including the popliteal hiatus) is inspected because this is a common location for loose bodies.

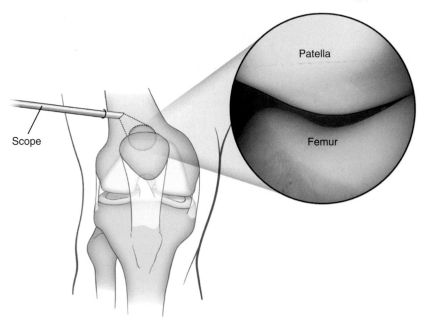

Figure 2-5. Visualization of the patellofemoral joint. *(From Miller MD, Chhabra AB, Hurwitz S, et al. [eds]. Orthopaedic Surgical Approaches. Philadelphia, Elsevier, 2008, p 487.)*

- Medial gutter
  - The scope is brought back up into the suprapatellar pouch and directed over the medial femoral condyle. A medial patellar plica (present in about 40% of knees) may be encountered. The knee can be flexed to better visualize the medial gutter.
- Intercondylar notch
  - The scope is directed back up into the suprapatellar pouch and then down to the intercondylar notch as the knee is taken from extension to flexion.
  - The surgeon should lower the scope tip (raise the camera) as the knee is flexed.
  - It is often helpful to use a shaver in the inferomedial portal to clear excessive fat pad and synovium during this maneuver.
  - The ligamentum mucosum is a synovial reflection that may obstruct complete visualization of the ACL and it can be easily removed with a shaver.
  - The ACL is inspected by directing the scope to view laterally and probing the ligament. The ACL is composed of two separate bundles that are often not distinct but can occasionally be recognized *(Fig. 2-6)*.
  - The PCL is evaluated. It is usually only possible to visualize the femoral insertion of the PCL on the medial femoral condyle

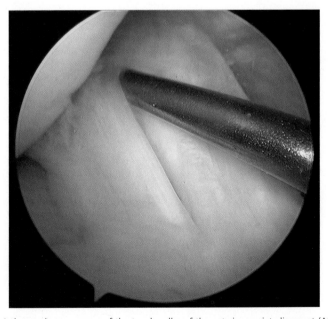

Figure 2-6. Arthroscopic appearance of the two bundles of the anterior cruciate ligament (ACL).

because the ACL hides most of this ligament. It is also enclosed in its own synovial sheath, so injuries may not be always appreciated. Indirect signs of PCL injury include pseudolaxity or sloppiness of the ACL, which is restored with an anterior drawer force.

- Meniscofemoral ligaments include the ligament of Humphry (anterior) and Wrisberg (posterior). These run from the posterior horn of the lateral meniscus to the respective portions of the PCL insertion.

- Modified Gillquist maneuver—allows access to the posterior knee through the intercondylar notch *(Fig. 2-7)*.

  ▸ Posteromedial: With the knee in 90-degree flexion, the scope sheath with blunt obturator is inserted through the inferolateral portal and along the wall of the medial femoral condyle until it "pops" into the back of the knee. The scope is then introduced and rotated to visualize the posteromedial joint. A spinal needle can be introduced (watch for the saphenous nerve and vein) and a portal can be established.

  ▸ Posterolateral: With the knee in 90-degree flexion, the scope sheath with blunt obturator is inserted through the inferomedial portal and along the wall of the lateral femoral

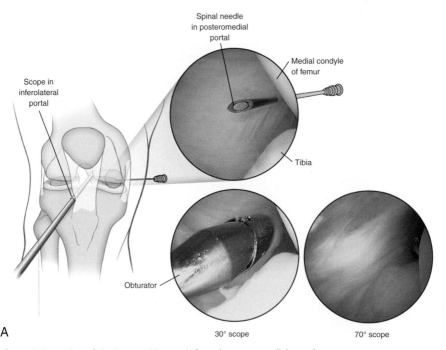

Figure 2-7. A. View of the intercondylar notch from the posteromedial portal.

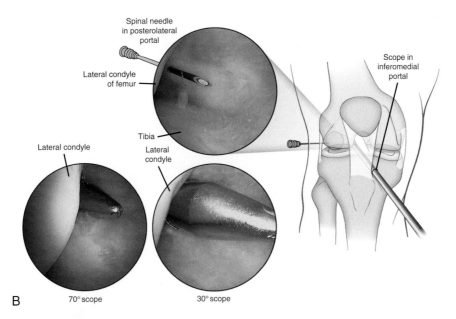

Figure 2.7—cont'd. **B.** View of the intercondylar notch from the posterolateral portal. *(From Miller MD, Chhabra AB, Hurwitz S, et al. [eds]. Orthopaedic Surgical Approaches. Philadelphia, Elsevier, 2008, pp 488-489.)*

condyle until it "pops" into the back of the knee. The scope is then introduced and rotated to visualize the posterolateral joint. A spinal needle is then introduced anterior to the biceps (to avoid the common peroneal nerve) and a portal can be established.

- **Medial compartment**
  - The arthroscope is moved from the intercondylar notch medially as the knee is extended and a valgus force is applied *(Fig. 2-8)*. The surgeon can apply this stress with the foot resting on his hip or an assistant can apply the force. The knee may need to be slightly flexed or the foot externally rotated to allow improved access.

  - The medial meniscus is carefully inspected and probed. It is helpful to consider the meniscus in zones as described by Cooper (Peripheral/Middle/Central and Posterior/Body/Anterior).

  - If a medial meniscal tear is present, determine (by probing) the location, size, and stability of the tear.

  - The articular surfaces are carefully examined for any chondral injuries. Palpation of the surfaces with a probe is carried out and documented. Lesions can be partial- or full-thickness injuries, focal or diffuse. Careful characterization, to include the size of the lesions, will guide treatment decisions.

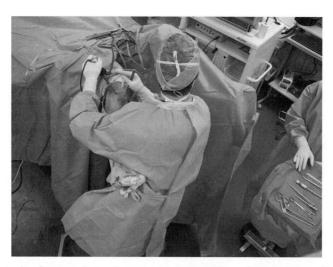

Figure 2-8. A valgus force is applied to allow easier visualization of the medial compartment. *(From Miller MD, Sekiya J. Sports Medicine. Core Knowledge in Orthopaedics. Philadelphia, Elsevier, 2006, p 26.)*

- Lateral compartment

  - The arthroscope is moved from the intercondylar notch laterally as the knee is placed in a figure-4 position *(Fig. 2-9)*. It is necessary for the surgeon to keep the scope focused on the anterior edge of the lateral femoral condyle as the knee is positioned and then it is swept into the lateral compartment. This maneuver requires some practice to master.

  - The lateral meniscus is carefully inspected and probed. Again, all tears are characterized by location, extent, size, and stability. Note that there is a normal hiatus, created by the traversing

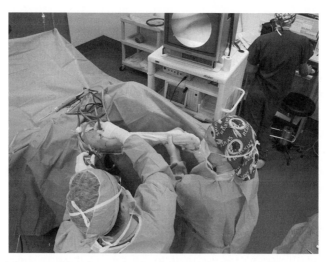

Figure 2-9. A figure-4 position allows easier visualization of the lateral compartment. *(From Miller MD, Sekiya J. Sports Medicine. Core Knowledge in Orthopaedics. Philadelphia, Elsevier, 2006, p 26.)*

popliteus tendon, at the junction of the posterior horn and body of the lateral meniscus.

■ Articular surfaces are probed and inspected and chondral injuries are characterized.

Common Knee Arthroscopic Procedures

Partial Meniscectomy (CPT 29881)

This is the most commonly performed procedure in all of orthopedics. It involves removal of an unrepairable meniscus tear using a combination of baskets and shavers *(Fig. 2-10)*. The tear is visualized, characterized, and then, if not repairable, it is removed. Removal of the minimal amount of meniscus possible will reduce the inherent risk of late arthrosis.

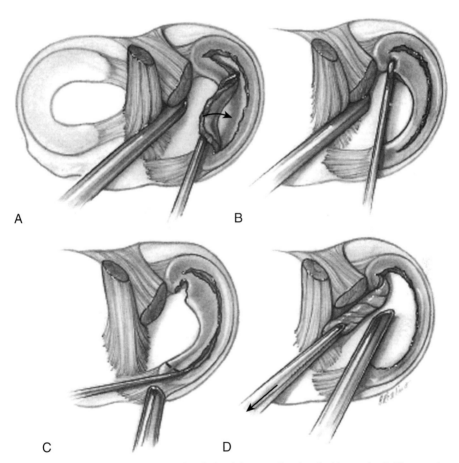

A   B

C   D

Figure 2-10. Partial meniscectomy. **A.** The displaced fragment is reduced with a probe. **B.** The posterior attachment is nearly transected under direct visualization with a biter. **C.** The anterior attachment is similarly transected. **D.** The fragment is grasped in line with the bulk of the meniscus and avulsed to remove. *(From Miller MD. Textbook of Arthroscopy. Philadelphia, Elsevier, 2004, p 511.)*

Meniscal Repair (CPT 29882)

This is recommended for all displaceable peripheral meniscal tears that have the potential for healing. A variety of techniques have been described including open (less popular except in combination with multiple ligament reconstruction), outside-in (also not as popular and uses spinal needles to introduce suture from outside the knee and through the meniscus), inside-out (uses special cannulas to pass suture on long needles ideally in a vertical mattress fashion) *(Fig. 2-11)*, and all-inside (a variety of implants have been developed for this purpose; the newest generation implants are "tensionable" *(Figs. 2-12 to 2-17)*.

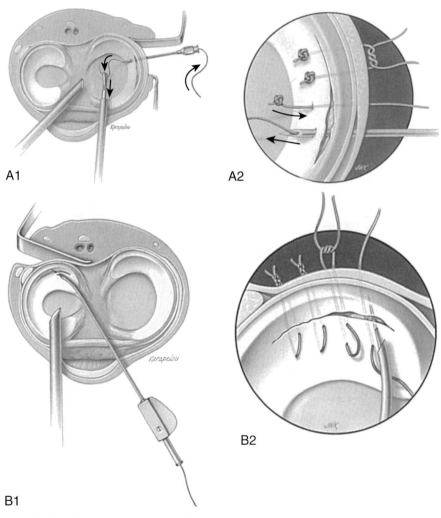

A1 A2

B1 B2

Figure 2-11. A. Outside-in meniscal repair. **A1.** Suture placement through a spinal needle. **A2.** "Mulberry knots" are tied to secure the repair. **B.** Inside-out meniscal repair. **B1.** Long needles are placed through cannulas. **B2.** Following suture placement, knots are tied over the joint capsule. *(From Miller MD. Review of Orthopaedics, 5th ed. Philadelphia, Elsevier, 2008, pp 255-256.)*

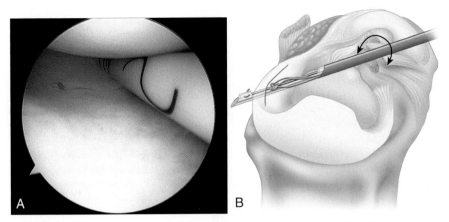

Figure 2-12. A and **B**. All-inside meniscal repair with FasT-Fix device. Use the needle to pierce the meniscus, crossing the tear site and then the meniscocapsular junction. *(From Miller MD. Operative Techniques: Sports Knee Surgery. Philadelphia, Elsevier, 2008, p 133.)*

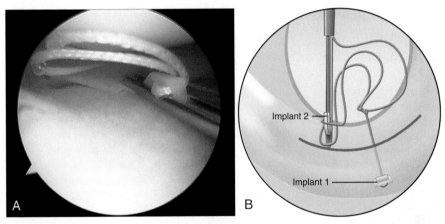

Figure 2-13. A and **B**. All-inside meniscal repair with FasT-Fix device. For the second implant, reposition the needle approximately 4 to 5 mm from the first implant. *(From Miller MD. Operative Techniques: Sports Knee Surgery. Philadelphia, Elsevier, 2008, p 133.)*

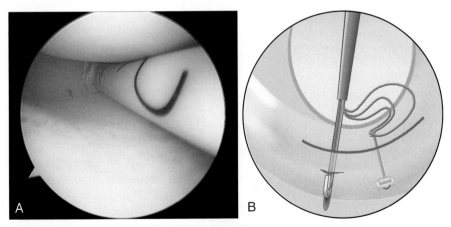

Figure 2-14. A and **B**. All-inside meniscal repair with FasT-Fix device. For the second implant, advance the needle through the tear and the meniscocapsular junction as before. *(From Miller MD. Operative Techniques: Sports Knee Surgery. Philadelphia, Elsevier, 2008, p 134.)*

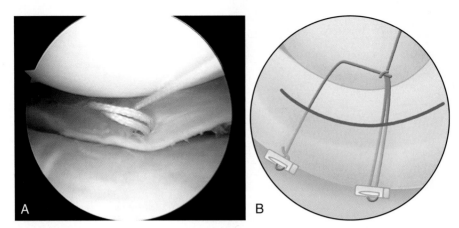

Figure 2-15. **A** and **B.** All-inside meniscal repair with FasT-Fix device. After crossing the meniscocapsular junction, oscillate the needle 5 to 10 degrees to deploy the second device. *(From Miller MD. Operative Techniques: Sports Knee Surgery. Philadelphia, Elsevier, 2008, p 134.)*

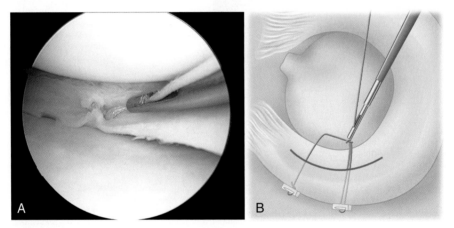

Figure 2-16. All-inside meniscal repair with FasT-Fix device. **A.** Holding the suture taut, advance the knot pusher and tighten the knot on top of the meniscal surface to reduce the tear **(B)**. *(From Miller MD. Operative Techniques: Sports Knee Surgery. Philadelphia, Elsevier, 2008, p 135.)*

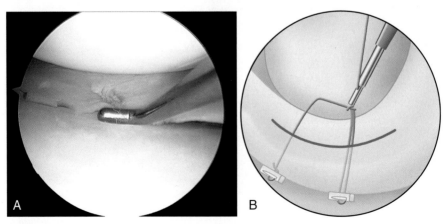

Figure 2-17. **A** and **B.** All-inside meniscal repair with FasT-Fix device. Cut the suture to finish the repair. *(From Miller MD. Operative Techniques: Sports Knee Surgery. Philadelphia, Elsevier, 2008, p 135.)*

Arthroscopic Synovectomy (CPT 29876)

Removal of part or all of the synovium can range from plica excision to a complete synovectomy. The latter is often required for diffuse pigmented villonodular synovitis (PVNS) and rheumatoid arthritis and requires the use of additional portals. An arthroscopic complete synovectomy through standard, superior, and posterior portals can be as effective as an open synovectomy. The arthroscope and shaver are introduced through a variety of portals and all synovium is systematically removed *(Figs. 2-18 and 2-19)*.

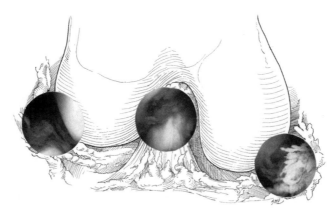

Figure 2-18. Arthroscopic appearance of diffuse PVNS. *(From Miller MD, Osborne JR, Warner JJP, et al. MRI-Arthroscopy Correlative Atlas. Philadelphia, Elsevier, 1997, p 38.)*

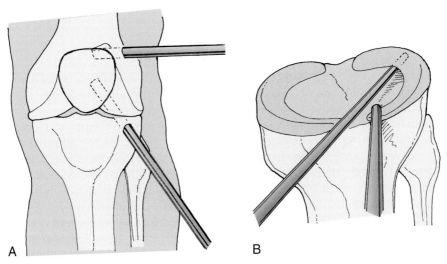

Figure 2-19. Steps for arthroscopic synovectomy. **A.** Suprapatellar pouch. **B.** Perimeniscal areas.

(Continued)

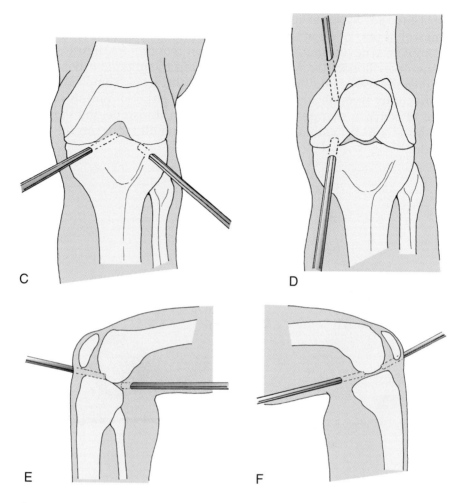

Figure 2-19—cont'd. C. Intercondylar notch, **D.** Switching portals. **E.** Posterolateral. **F.** Posteromedial. *(From Miller MD, Howard RF, and Plancher KD. Surgical Atlas of Sports Medicine. Philadelphia, Elsevier, 2003, pp 39-40.)*

Articular Cartilage Procedures (CPT 29877, 29879, 29866)

These procedures are designed to address focal traumatic cartilage defects. They include shaving chondroplasty, microfracture, osteochondral plug transfer, autologous chondrocyte implantation, and allografts. All of the procedures begin with débridement of the edges of the lesions and documenting the size of the defect. Microfracture, which is a so-called *marrow stimulation procedure*, includes debriding the base of the lesion (removing the calcified cartilage layer) and then making a series of holes in the subchondral bone using a specially designed awl *(Fig. 2-20)*. Osteochondral plug transfer (sometimes named for the equipment used— OATS (Arthrex, Naples, FL), mosaicplasty (Smith & Nephew, Andover, MA) or COR (Depuy-Mitek, Raynham, MA)) involves taking a cylinder of bone and cartilage from an area of the knee that has the lowest contact pressures

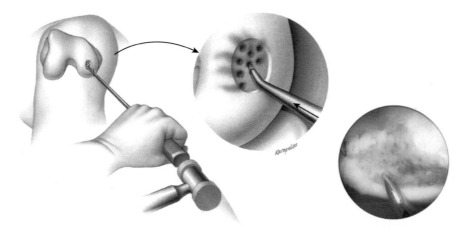

Figure 2-20. Microfracture uses special awls to penetrate the subchondral bone approximately 4 mm. *(From Miller MD. Atlas of chondral injury treatment. Op Tech Orthop 7:289-293, 1997.)*

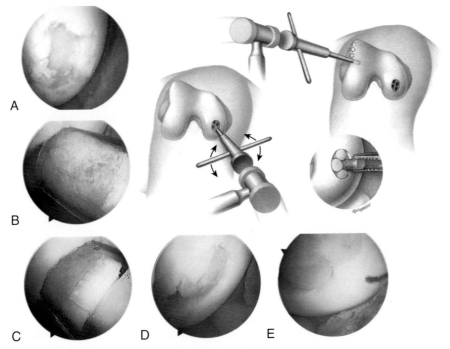

Figure 2-21. Osteochondral plug transfer. **A** and **B.** Drill perpendicular to the joint surface. **C.** Deliver the plug. **D.** Drill second plug. **E.** Completed plug transfer. *(From Miller MD. Atlas of chondral injury treatment. Op Tech Orthop 7:289-293, 1997.)*

(such as the superolateral trochlea) and transferring this plug into a specially prepared recipient site in the defect *(Fig. 2-21)*. Autologous chondrocyte implantation (ACI) is a two-stage procedure in which a small amount of uninvolved cartilage is harvested and sent to the lab to culture chondrocytes. These are then injected into the defect and help with a patch of periosteum that is sewn in place *(Fig. 2-22)*. Allograft plug transfer is very

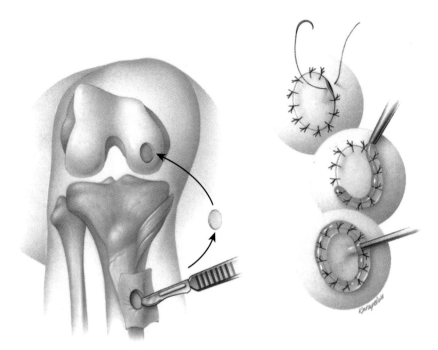

Figure 2-22. Autologous chondrocyte implantation. *(From Miller MD. Atlas of chondral injury treatment. Op Tech Orthop 7:289-293, 1997.)*

similar to osteochondral plug transfer described earlier, but larger defects can be addressed with this technique that utilizes sized allograft tissue.

Anterior Cruciate Ligament (ACL) Reconstruction (CPT 29888)

This procedure involves harvesting a hamstring (semitendinosus and gracilis) or central one third of the bone-patellar tendon-bone graft and passing it through drill holes to replace the torn ACL *(Fig. 2-23)*.

Complications

- Iatrogenic chondromalacia
  - Likely under-reported, this complication can be minimized with careful handling of the arthroscope and instruments, careful portal placement, and adequate visualization. Instruments should never be "forced" into the knee. In teaching centers, "resident malacia" should be discouraged.

- Hemarthrosis
  - Meticulous technique and visualization following tourniquet release can minimize this uncommon complication. Particular care should be taken with procedures such as a lateral release. A postoperative drain, even when removed in the recovery room, can sometimes be helpful.

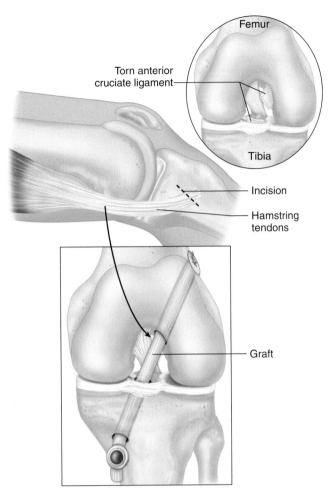

Figure 2-23. Anterior cruciate ligament reconstruction.

- **Infection**
  - Although this occurs in only less than 1% of knee arthroscopies, it can be a devastating complication. Strict sterile technique should be maintained at all times. Although prophylactic antibiotic use is usually not recommended for simple arthroscopy, it should be used for more complicated procedures. *Staphylococcus aureus* and *Staphylococcus epidermidis* are common pathogens and may be difficult to recognize early on. Aspiration, laboratory studies (including erythrocyte sedimentation rate [ESR] and C-reactive protein [CRP]) and systemic symptoms should be evaluated. Urgent irrigation and débridement (and usually synovectomy) are required for an established infection and can be done arthroscopically.

- Arthrofibrosis
  - This is unusual after a simple arthroscopy, but it can occur with procedures such as ACL reconstruction and multiple ligament reconstructions, especially if full motion is not present preoperatively.
- Anesthesia complications
  - These are present for all surgeries, and the complications are similar.
  - Regional blocks are commonly given for several arthroscopic procedures and these have their own inherent risks.
- Deep vein thrombosis
  - Certain risk factors (obesity, elderly patients, smoking history, use of birth control pills, clotting disorders, prolonged tourniquet times, etc.) have a cumulative effect on DVT risk. Prophylaxis should be considered for high-risk patients.
  - A high index of suspicion is appropriate with postoperative patients who present with calf tightness, pain, and swelling. Noninvasive studies (e.g., ultrasonography) should be considered if there is any question.
- Neurovascular injury
  - This is an unusual complication but it highlights the importance of proper technique, particularly in creating posterior portals and in placing the arthroscope and/or instruments posteriorly.
- Instrument failure
  - This is a rare complication but it can occur. Instruments should be serviced regularly. If an instrument breaks, the broken pieces must be identified and removed *(Fig. 2-24)*.

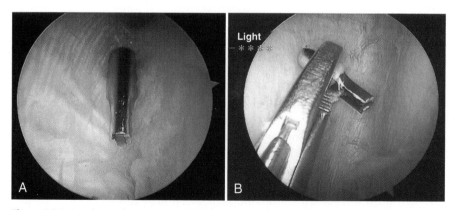

Figure 2-24. A and B. Broken grasper.

- Synovial cutaneous fistula
  - This is also a rare complication and is usually managed by immobilizing the knee in full extension for several days. If it persists, it may require formal excision, débridement, and closure.

REFERENCES

Baer GS and Sekiya JK. Knee arthroscopy—the basics. In Miller MD, Cole BJ, Cosgarea AJ, and Sekiya JK (eds). *Sports Knee Surgery*, Philadelphia, Elsevier, 2008; pp 23–39.

Cooper DE, Arnoaky SP, and Warren RF. Arthroscopic meniscal repair. *Clin Sports Med* 1990; 9(3):589–608.

Diduch DR, Shen FR, Ong BC, et al. Knee: Diagnostic arthroscopy. In Miller MD and Cole BJ (eds). *Textbook of Arthroscopy*, Philadelphia, Elsevier, 2004; pp 471–487.

Ishibashi Y and Yamamoto Y. The history of arthroscopy. In Miller MD and Cole BJ (eds). *Textbook of Arthroscopy*, Philadelphia, Elsevier, 2004; pp 3–7.

Jackson RW. History of arthroscopy. In McGinty JB (ed). *Operative Arthroscopy*, New York, Raven Press, 1991; pp 1–4.

Miller MD. Knee and lower leg. In Miller MD, Chhabra AB, Hurwitz S, et al. (eds). *Orthopaedic Surgical Approaches*, Philadelphia, Elsevier, 2008; pp 423–490.

Miller MD, Cole BJ, Cosgarea AJ, and Sekiya JK. *Sports Knee Surgery*, Philadelphia, Elsevier, 2008; 23–142, 165–220, 277–298.

Miller MD, Howard RF, and Plancher KD. *Surgical Atlas of Sports Medicine*, Philadelphia, Elsevier, 2003.

Miller MD and Sekiya JK. Knee arthroscopy. In Miller MD and Sekiya JK (eds). *Core Knowledge in Orthopaedics: Sports Medicine*, Philadelphia, Elsevier, 2006; pp 22–26.

Ong BC, Shen FH, Musahl V, et al. Knee: Patient positioning, portal placement, and normal arthroscopy anatomy. In Miller MD and Cole BJ (eds). *Textbook of Arthroscopy*, Philadelphia, Elsevier, 2004; pp 463–469.

CHAPTER 3

Hip Arthroscopy

Sanaz Hariri and Marc R. Safran

History and Background

- First described in 1931 by Burman in a cadaver study. However, he declared "that it is impossible to separate the head of the femur from the acetabulum ... It is manifestly impossible to insert a needle between the head of the femur and the acetabulum. One cannot, therefore, hope to see the acetabular fossa." He was only able to see a part of the femoral head, the junction of the femoral head and neck, and the femoral neck.
- Takagi was the first to report on the clinical application of hip arthroscopy in 1939.
- Development of improved traction devices and instrumentation eventually made hip arthroscopy more versatile.
- Initial slow development but recently rapid increase in enthusiasm for hip arthroscopy since the 1990s
- Technically more demanding than arthroscopy of other joints with a longer learning curve even for experienced surgeons
- Challenges:
  - Thick capsule, muscle envelope, and periarticular ligaments make distraction difficult.
  - Convex femoral head and deeply recessed in a bony acetabulum makes joint entry difficult.
  - Curvilinear articulating surface makes navigation difficult.
  - Deep joint due to periarticular muscles and soft tissues, as well as the thick capsule, makes maneuverability within the joint difficult.
  - Offers shorter recovery times and quicker return to activity than do open procedures
  - Many injuries now addressed arthroscopically had been largely undiagnosed and untreated until recently.

Preoperative Workup

- Key to success is careful patient selection
- First determine if the source of pain is intra-articular.

- Hallmarks of intra-articular hip pathology:
  - Groin pain usually increasing with activity but largely unresponsive to conservative treatment (e.g., ice, rest, nonsteroidal anti-inflammatory drugs [NSAIDs], and physical therapy)
  - Relatively well-tolerated activities: motion in a straight plane, activity on level surfaces
  - Poorly tolerated activities: torsional/twisting activity, prolonged hip flexion (e.g., sitting), rising from a seated position (causes pain/catching), activity on inclines
  - Presence of mechanical symptoms (clicking, catching, locking, or giving way/buckling) preoperatively is a favorable prognostic indicator for hip arthroscopy for any diagnosis except degenerative arthritis
  - A positive McCarthy sign is significantly correlated with intra-articular pathology (with both hips fully flexed: the pain is reproduced by extending the affected hip in external and/or internal rotation)
  - Relief of pain with an injection of an anesthetic into the hip joint can help distinguish between intra- and extra-articular pathology
- Must rule out referred pain from lumbar or sacral areas, genitourinary tract, gastrointestinal system, and abdominal wall
- Cautionary signs: ill-defined symptoms or examination findings, unreasonable expectations, a stiff hip
- Radiographs
  - Plain films to look for osteophytes (make entry into the joint difficult), degenerative arthritis (indicator of poor prognosis), ossified and metallic loose bodies, anatomy of femoroacetabular impingement (FAI) and dysplasia *(Fig. 3-1)*
  - Conventional computed tomography (CT) and magnetic resonance imaging (MRI) lack sensitivity and specificity in diagnosing labral pathology.
  - Gadolinium arthrography combined with high resolution, thin-cut multiplaning MRA (MR arthrography) with small field of view (focus on the affected hip rather than on the pelvis) is best for assessing labral pathology *(Fig. 3-2)*.
  - 74% Sensitivity, 83% specificity, and 78% accuracy in diagnosing anterior labral pathology
- Hip dysplasia → increased incidence of labral, chondral, and ligamentum teres lesions *(Fig. 3-3)*
  - Shallow bony acetabulum (usually with hypertrophied labrum) → labrum playing an increased role in weight-bearing and joint

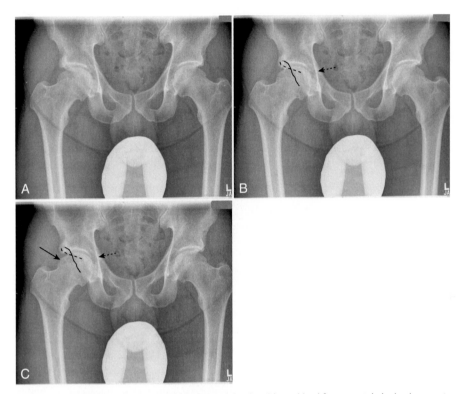

Figure 3-1. A. AP Pelvis of a 40-year-old male martial artist with combined femoroacetabular impingement. **B.** Shows the line for cross-over with the *solid line* being the posterior wall of the acetabulum and the *dashed line* outlining the anterior wall demonstrating the cranial retroversion of the acetabulum seen with pincer type of impingement. The *dashed arrow* demonstrating the floor of the acetabulum touches the ilioischial line, as seen with coxa profunda. **C.** Includes an *arrow* pointing at the cam lesion.

stability → exposure to greater joint reaction and weight-bearing forces → increased risk of labrum inversion and tearing

■ Reduced chondral surface area → increased contact forces → overload leads to chondral wear as well as acute fragmentation and early degeneration (edge loading)

■ Lateral subluxation of the femoral head → elongation or hypertrophy of the ligamentum teres → ligament may become entrapped or undergoes a partial or complete degenerative rupture

■ Presence of dysplasia is not itself a poor prognostic indicator (as previously thought); response to treatment is dictated by the nature of the intra-articular pathology.

● One must consider whether large bony dysmorphisms (e.g., FAI and dysplasia) causing labral and chondral pathology are best treated with osteotomies or other open bony procedures to address the underlying pathology.

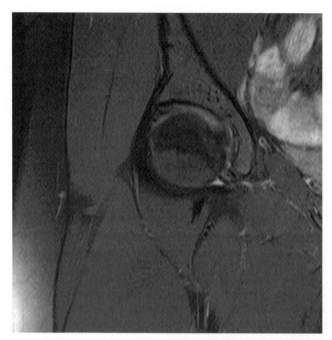

Figure 3-2. MRI gadolinium arthrogram—coronal view demonstrating a labral tear.

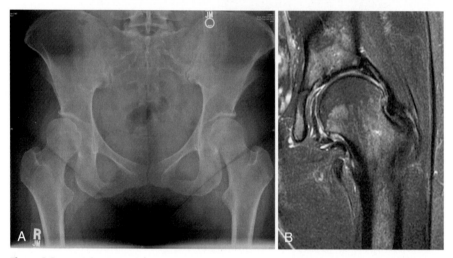

Figure 3-3. A. An AP pelvis of a patient with dysplasia. B. An MRI showing large labrum in dysplasia.

Indications

- Loose bodies (e.g., from trauma, synovial chondromatosis, osteoarthritis, and Legg-Calvé-Perthes disease): the clearest indication for hip arthroscopy
- Classifications: ossified versus nonossified; osteoocartilaginous, cartilaginous, fibrous, or foreign

- Labral lesions/tears
    - Controversy over etiology of labral tears: are they predominantly the result of bony impingement (the prevailing theory) or do they happen independently due to dynamic load or torque (e.g., sudden twisting or pivoting motions) as in the knee joint (McCarthy)
    - Typically present with moderate-to-severe, sharp and/or dull activity-related groin pain (e.g., pain with walking and pivoting); most patients also have night pain and painful mechanical locking
    - Pathology often overlooked: mean time from onset of symptoms to diagnosis is 21 months; mean number of health-care providers seen before definitive diagnosis is 3.3.
    - >80% of patients with atraumatic onset of symptoms related to labral tears have associated underlying bony pathology (FAI, dysplasia).
    - Positive impingement test: axial force with hip flexion-adduction-internal rotation → shearing and compression forces on the labrum → pain
    - Most tears are anterior or anterolateral and occur at the relatively avascular inner portion of the tissue.
    - May have bucket-handle tear after a posterior hip dislocation that may block closed reduction
    - Question if labral tears contribute to the progression of hip osteoarthritis (OA) or if labral débridement/repair alters the natural history: still need studies
    - >50% of all labral tears have associated chondral damage: damaged labrum → joint fluid is pumped under the acetabular chondral surface with repetitive loading → delamination of the articular cartilage → fluid burrows beneath the subchondral bone → forms a subchondral cyst.
- Chondral lesions of the acetabulum or femoral head
    - Vast majority occur in the anterior quadrants of the acetabulum *(Fig. 3-4)*
    - Most frequently associated with a labral tear
    - Over years, flap lesions progress via a delamination mechanism.
    - "Lateral impact injury" can occur after a blow to the greater trochanter → energy and load transferred to the joint surface
    - Grade of chondral lesion is most predictive of surgical outcome.

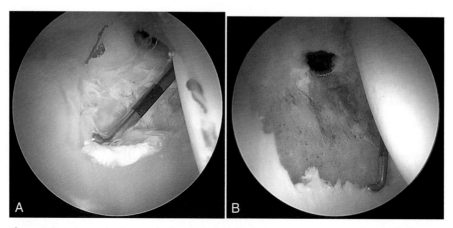

Figure 3-4. Arthroscopic photograph of a 21-year-old baseball player with FAI of the right hip. **A.** Shows chondral delamination of the anterolateral acetabular articular cartilage. **B.** Demonstrates this chondral lesion after chondroplasty.

- Chondral loss (especially of the femoral head) is poor prognostic indicator for arthroscopy.

- Ligamentum teres rupture: an increasingly recognized source of hip pain; third most common pathology diagnosed in athletes undergoing hip arthroscopy *(Fig. 3-5)*

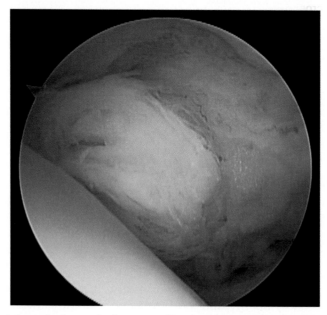

Figure 3-5. Arthroscopic photograph of a 32-year-old male with hip pain as a result of a tear of the ligamentum teres. The femoral head is to the left and the cotyloid fossa is on the right.

- Can occur after a twisting injury even without hip subluxation/ dislocation

- Atraumatic degenerative cases associated with osteoarthritis and hip dysplasia

- Imaging and physical examination findings not very specific

- Usually present with groin pain and mechanical symptoms

- Patients may avoid extending the hip while walking.

- **Degenerative disease: perform arthroscopy with caution**
  - Patients with degenerative changes apparent on plain hip radiographs are significantly more likely to have poor clinical results following hip arthroscopy than those with normal hip radiographs.

- **Persistent pain following hip dislocation**
  - 79% to 92% of traumatic hip dislocation patients who underwent arthroscopy were found to have osteochondral loose bodies within the joint despite some having no evidence of loose bodies on radiographs and CT scans.

  - In one study, all 14 hip dislocation patients had labral tears and chondral defects seen on arthroscopy; 79% had partial or complete tears of the ligamentum teres.

- **Osteonecrosis/avascular necrosis (AVN): for early cases to address concomitant pathology (e.g., loose bodies, synovitis, chondral flaps, and labral tears) and to more precisely stage AVN during the workup for a possible revascularization procedure**
  - Not successful for end-stage disease with femoral head collapse

  - Best results in lower-grade lesions where loose bodies are found and removed

  - During core decompression: used for intra-articular observation to ensure no joint penetration and to ensure that the core track is within the avascular zone

- **Synovial disease (e.g., inflammatory arthritis, synovial chondromatosis, pigmented villonodular synovitis [PVNS])**
  - Palliative

  - For diagnostic biopsy

  - Cannot do complete synovectomy arthroscopically

  - Results partially dependent on integrity of articular cartilage

- **Femoroacetabular impingement (FAI) described by Ganz**
  - Cam impingement: when a nonspherical femoral head abuts the anterior acetabulum, particularly with hip flexion
    - ▸ Causes: poor head-neck offset, posttraumatic deformities, slipped capital femoral epiphysis (SCFE), femoral retrotorsion, coxa vara, femoral head AVN with flattening, sequelae of Legg-Calvé-Perthes disease
  - Pincer impingement: due to overcoverage of the acetabulum anteriorly or acetabular retroversion (see *Fig. 3-1*)
  - Causes: acetabular retroversion (global or cranial), coxa profunda, protrusio
  - Majority have combined cam and pincer impingement (see *Fig. 3-1C*)
  - Present with groin pain, especially when sitting for prolonged periods and crossing the symptomatic leg; positive impingement test (pain with maximum internal rotation and adduction with the hip flexed to 90 degrees)
  - Limited range of motion (ROM), particularly of internal rotation
  - FAI → repetitive microtrauma to the labrum at extremes of hip motion → labral and chondral lesions (see *Fig. 3-4*) → ?early-onset hip osteoarthritis
- **Atraumatic instability: capsular laxity with iliofemoral ligament deficiency**
  - Less common in the hip than in the shoulder because of the hip's intrinsic osseous stability
  - Not well delineated at this time
  - Associated with collagen vascular disorders (e.g., Ehlers-Danlos syndrome)
- **Irrigation and débridement (I&D) of a septic hip**
  - Contraindications to arthroscopic (versus open) treatment: longstanding or recurrent infection, osteomyelitis, particularly virulent bacteria, extracapsular abscess (should get a CT scan or MRI before arthroscopy to assess)
  - Can perform arthroscopic I&D of an infected total hip arthroplasty (THA) patient if: early diagnosis, components well fixed, a sensitive microorganism
- **Adhesive capsulitis: characterized by painful restricted ROM often with a precipitating event (e.g., a fall or twist), predilection for middle-aged women, radiographs usually normal**
- **Foreign bodies (e.g., bullets, broken trochanteric wire, acetabular screw that is backing out, broken guidewire fragment from cannulated screw fixation)**

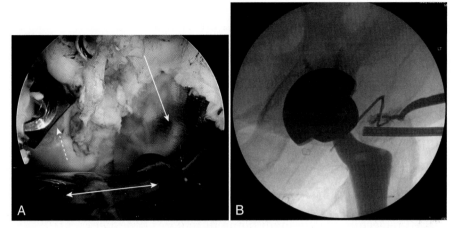

Figure 3-6. A. An arthroscopic view of the neck (*white arrow with double head*) and base of the metallic femoral head (*white arrow*) in a patient with a total hip arthroplasty with broken wire—*dashed arrow* points to clamp of broken wire. **B.** A fluoroscopic view of same patient during removal of the broken wire.

- Painful THAs (e.g., débridement of porous beads due to metal-on-metal corrosion at the head-neck junction; synovial biopsy to assess for infection when the hip aspiration is negative but clinical suspicion is high; débridement of scar tissue and adhesions, removal of broken or migrated wires) *(Fig. 3-6)*
  - Hip arthroscopy either successfully treated or directly led to successful treatment in 8 of 12 THA cases with persistent pain and a nondiagnostic standard workup
- Osteochondrosis dissecans: rarely in the hip, can remove the dissecate and then microfracture
- Pipkin fractures of the femoral head
- Crystalline hip arthropathy (gout and pseudogout): may present with extreme hip pain, difficult diagnosis if limited to the hip because patient may have a normal serum uric acid level with just a joint effusion on MRI
  - Arthroscopic treatment: copious lavage, mechanical crystal débridement, synovial biopsy for definitive diagnosis
- Chondral cyst: focal, compressible chondral elevation detected on hip arthroscopy in a Legg-Calvé-Perthes patient with persistent hip stiffness
  - Flocculent fluid released on incision of the cyst, the underlying chondral defect was microfractured → patient had immediate pain relief with continued painless ROM at 4-year follow-up
- Hereditary multiple exostoses with a lesion in the hip joint causing pain and limited ROM
- Giant-cell tumor of the ligamentum teres: a case report involving a 46-year-old woman with thigh/groin/buttock pain, full hip ROM, a positive impingement sign, and an MRI suggestive of a labral tear; tumor was successfully excised arthroscopically

- Pediatric hip condition, for example:
  - Legg-Calvé-Perthes disease (e.g., for loose bodies)
  - Developmental dysplasia of the hip (typically to address a labral tear after osteotomy to correct the underlying dysplasia)
  - Septic arthritis
  - Juvenile rheumatoid arthritis (RA)
  - Slipped capital femoral epiphysis to address:
    - Chondrolysis as a result of pin penetration of the cartilage during fixation
    - Osteonecrosis from damage to retinacular vessels
    - Chielectomy for residual bump at femoral head-neck junction that may be impeding hip motion or causing pain from impingement *(Fig. 3-7)*
- Possible indications for periacetabular osteotomy versus arthroscopy:
  - Moderate-to-severe hip dysplasia
  - Actual hip subluxation
  - Coxa valga greater than 140 degrees
  - Upsloping sourcil
- Intractable hip pain resistant to conservative treatment and intra-articular injection with negative radiographic workup but mechanical symptoms: arthroscopy facilitates diagnosis in 40% of these cases
- Extra-articular conditions

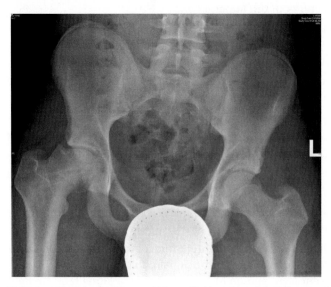

Figure 3-7. AP Pelvis radiograph of a 17-year-old boy with hip pain and limited range of motion with evidence of residuals of slipped capital femoral epiphysis.

- Snapping hip syndrome: three types

  ▸ External/lateral: most common type, caused by snapping of either posterior border of iliotibial band (ITB) or anterior border of gluteus maximus over greater trochanter when hip moves from extension to flexion

  ▸ Internal: painful snapping of iliopsoas tendon over the iliopectineal eminence, femoral head, or iliofemoral ligament

  • Arthroscopy better than open treatment: can eliminate snapping without nerve complications or weakness

  • 70% to 80% Associated with intra-articular pathology that can be addressed concomitantly with hip arthroscopy

  ▸ Intra-articular: caused by loose body/bodies in the joint (e.g., fracture fragment, piece of labrum, chondral flap), pain elicited by hip rotation

- Iliopsoas bursitis

- Greater trochanteric pain syndrome differential diagnosis:

  ▸ ITB tendonitis

  ▸ Trochanteric bursitis

  ▸ Avulsion of the gluteus medius ± minimus tendon (*Fig. 3-8*)

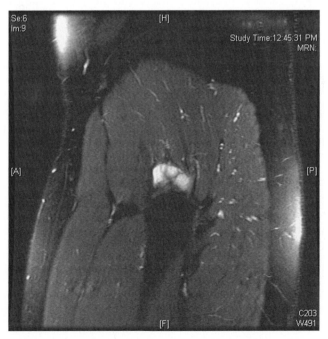

Figure 3-8. Sagittal T2 MRI demonstrating an avulsion of the gluteus medius in a 32-year-old male with acute onset of hip pain, 4 weeks prior to the MRI.

- Seen in 20% of women >65 years old undergoing THR
- Repair arthroscopically if failed rehabilitation for hip abductor weakness

Contraindications

- Open wounds, especially near portal placement sites
- Systemic disease
- Severe restrictions to joint entry (e.g., marked capsular restriction, arthrofibrosis, ankylosis, dense heterotopic ossification [HO])
- Osteopenia/osteoporosis to the degree that the bone is unable to withstand the necessary traction forces
- Bone tumors close to the joint
- Sepsis with osteomyelitis or abscess formation
- Reflex dystrophia
- Risk factors for joint fluid extravasation: recent acetabular fracture, extensive capsular rupture
- Morbid obesity (instrumentation may not be long enough to access the joint or strong enough to maneuver within the joint)
- Advanced coxarthrosis
- Caution in AVN because the fluid pressure and the traction may further compromise the blood supply to the femoral head

Preoperative Considerations

- Complete routine preoperative protocol: i.e., consultation with appropriate medical, cardiology, and anesthesia colleagues; review of history, physical examination, radiographs, and lab tests; review consent form with patient and sign the correct joint in the preoperative holding area
- Anesthesia
  - Almost always general anesthesia because complete muscle relaxation via a neuromuscular blockade is required so that one may use the least amount of force necessary to achieve sufficient joint distraction
  - May be performed under epidural anesthesia with adequate motor block to achieve required hip distraction
  - Can consider supplemental lumbar plexus block for perioperative analgesia

Relevant Anatomy

- Hip joint: a large ball-and-socket diarthrodial or synovial joint ~0.5 cm distal to the middle third of the inguinal ligament
- Two compartments
  - Central compartment: the weight-bearing part of the hip joint (corresponding joint surfaces of the acetabulum and femoral head), intracapsular and intra-articular
  - Peripheral compartment: the non–weight-bearing part of the femoral head and the femoral neck up to the capsule insertion, intracapsular but extra-articular, free-floating loose bodies can hide here
- Femoral head: two thirds of a sphere, average head diameter at the equatorial plane: 48.3 mm (range 40 to 58 mm), flattened at the area of greatest load on the acetabulum
- Acetabulum: a hemisphere with a peripheral horseshoe–shaped articular surface
  - nonarticular fossa ovalis inferomedially
  - typically oriented in ~45 degrees of abduction and 15 to 20 degrees of anteversion
- Labrum: triangular fibrocartilage that runs circumferentially around the acetabular perimeter to the base of the fovea where the transverse acetabular ligament completes it by extending across the acetabular notch
- Vascularized only on its outermost capsular perimeter
- Contains free nerve endings (proprioceptors and nociceptors)
- Some functions:
  - Provides negative intra-articular pressure in the joint
  - Acts as a tension band to limit expansion during gait when the loading leads to motion of the anterior and posterior columns
  - Elevated role in stability and weight-bearing in dysplastic patients
  - Functions as a seal/O ring to maintain synovial fluid in the central compartment, lubricating the joint and providing nutrition to the articular cartilage
- Ligamentum teres: intra-articular but extracapsular, extends from the transverse acetabular ligament to the fovea of the femoral head, large ligament, main blood supply to the femoral head before 14 years of age but unclear function after that age, unclear stabilizing effect on the joint, tightens in external rotation

- Capsule
    - Ligaments are capsular thickenings.
    - Does not attach to the labrum
    - Proximally: covers the labrum
    - Distally: attaches to the intertrochanteric line on the anterior femoral neck; attaches just proximal to the intertrochanteric crest on the posterior femoral neck → therefore you can see more of the anterior than the posterior femoral neck arthroscopically
    - Anteriorly: consists primarily of the strong Y ligament of Bigelow (iliofemoral ligament, strongest ligament in the human body) which resists hip extension and external rotation
    - Anterolaterally: pubofemoral ligament (restricts hip abduction)
    - Posteriorly: Ischiofemoral ligament (restricts internal rotation)
- Zona orbicularis: a ligament around the neck of the femur at the base of the femoral head, may help maintain the femoral head within the acetabulum, resists distraction forces
- Fibers of Weitbrecht are medial and lateral synovial folds in the peripheral compartment, "the lighthouse of the peripheral compartment," retinacular branches of the medial femoral circumflex artery pass deep to it to reach the femoral head, often incorrectly referred to as the "ligament of Weitbrecht" (which is in the elbow).
- Psoas bursa: communicates with the anterior hip joint in 20% of patients.
- Surrounding neurovascular structures: femoral nerve and artery anteriorly; lateral femoral cutaneous nerve (LFCN) anterolaterally (usually divides into 3 or more branches at the level of the anterior portal); sciatic nerve, and gluteal vessels posteriorly
- Anterior capsule most relaxed with hip flexion; posterior capsule most relaxed in external rotation; capsule overall tightest with full hip extension

Position

- Choice based on surgeon preference and training
- Supine (popularized by Byrd)
    - Pros: familiar orientation of the joint; can use a standard fracture table with a standard perineal post for traction; ease of conversion to open anterior or anterolateral approach
    - Cons: pannus in obese patients can interfere with instrument movement
- Lateral decubitus (popularized by Glick)
    - Pros: in obese patients the pannus and buttock drop away from the operative field, increasing maneuverability; easier access to posterior

portal (particularly valuable in the presence of a large anterolateral osteophyte blocking portal access); familiarity with the position for arthroplasty surgeons who use the lateral decubitus position

■ Cons: more time needed to position the patient; must either manipulate the standard fracture table or use special traction devices attached to a standard operating table

Equipment

● Typical room set-up *(Figs. 3-9 and 3-10)*

■ On the operative side (if supine) OR posterior to the patient (if lateral decubitus): surgeon, scrub nurse, backtable with instruments, and sterile Mayo stand with the most commonly used instruments (placed over the patient's torso)

■ On the contralateral side (if supine) OR anterior to the patient (if lateral decubitus): arthroscopic video tower monitor, fluoroscopy screen (although this can be at the foot of the table instead)

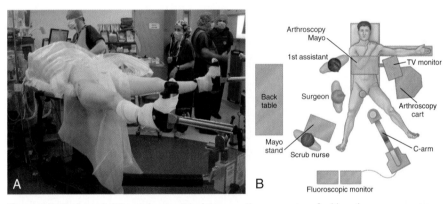

Figure 3-9. Photograph (**A**) and drawing (**B**) of the operating room set-up for hip arthroscopy.

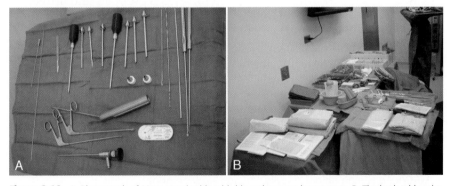

Figure 3-10. **A.** Photograph of Mayo stand table with hip arthroscopy instruments. **B.** The back table prior to draping of a hip arthroscopy patient.

- Table
  - For the supine position:
    - Patient supine on a standard fracture table
    - Abduct the contralateral hip (makes room for the C-arm between the legs)
  - For the lateral position:
    - Patient lateral decubitus with operative hip superior (protect neurovascular structures in axilla)
    - Pad the contralateral leg (special care to protect the peroneal nerve at the fibular head)
    - Fracture table, but must reposition the perineal post and traction device OR
    - Standard operating table with commercially available distraction device
    - Swing the C-arm under the table for anteroposterior views if needed
  - Tensiometer can monitor the traction forces (senior author [MRS] has not found this to be useful)
  - Perineal post: well-padded against the operative leg's medial thigh
    - Provides countertraction for hip distraction
    - Large surface area distributes traction forces to protect the perineum
    - Lateralizes the hip to optimize the distraction vector
- Large C-arm fluoroscopy
  - To confirm necessary distraction
  - To assist with portal placement if necessary
  - Must be sterilely draped if used after the leg is prepped and draped
- Arthroscope ("scope")
  - 30-degree scope: best for viewing the central acetabulum and femoral head and superior acetabular fossa, useful in the peripheral compartment
  - 70-degree scope: best for viewing the acetabular labrum, acetabular rim, anterior capsule, inferior acetabular fossa, most peripheral aspects of the joint
- Fluid pump optional (senior author uses gravity)
- 16-Gauge 6-inch spinal needle for portal placement

- Nitinol guidewire (threaded through the spinal needle)
- Extra-long cannulas (4.5, 5.0, and 5.5 mm) with blunt and sharp obturators/trochars (senior author does not use the sharp obturators/trochars)
- Arthroscopic probe (rigid and flexible) to palpate and manipulate structures
- Curved instruments to maneuver around the femoral head
- Slotted cannulas for curved instruments: the slot is one third of the cannula pipe, the sharp tip of the instrument should always be inside the slot to prevent iatrogenic injury
- Electrothermal device(s)
- Long motorized shaver(s) and burr(s)
- Modified meniscal biters—straight and back biters
- Long, narrow curettes
- Loose body retrievers
- Long, narrow rongeurs
- Straight and angled picks for microfracture
- Suture passing and retrieving instruments

Portals *(Fig. 3-11)*

- Palpable landmarks
  - Anterior superior iliac spine (ASIS)
  - Greater trochanter

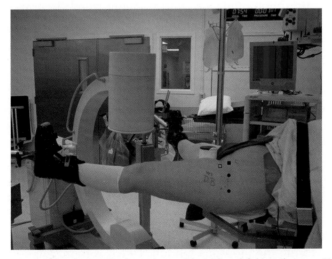

Figure 3-11. Intraoperative photograph of a patient positioned for a left hip arthroscopy. Marked on the skin are the patient's greater trochanter and an outline of the anterior superior iliac spine. The *two black circles* represent the anterolateral and posterolateral portals, whereas the *open black square* represents the position for the modified anterior portal—7 cm distal and medial to the anterolateral portal at a 45-degree angle. The complete *black square* represents the standard anterior portal, at the junction of the anterior superior iliac spine and greater trochanter.

- Femoral pulse
- Pubic symphysis
- Femoral shaft

- The same three basic portals for central compartment hip arthroscopy are used by most surgeons for the supine and lateral decubitus positions: anterolateral, anterior, and posterolateral.
- Anterolateral (AL)/anterior paratrochanteric portal
  - Start at the superoanterior margin of the greater trochanter → pass through the gluteus medius and minimus muscles → enter hip close to femoral head with long end of needle bevel pointed away from the femoral head
  - Usually the first portal is established because it is easiest to access, is reproducible, and puts the surrounding neurovascular structures at less risk
  - Usually performed under fluoroscopic visualization
  - Can be repositioned onto the anterior femoral neck to access the peripheral compartment
  - All other portals are established under direct arthroscopic visualization.
  - Occasionally this portal is made after entering the peripheral compartment. To help reduce risk of injury to the labrum, this technique allows for making the portal while passing the spinal needle (and then guidewire and trochar) from the proposed anterolateral portal under arthroscopic visualization from the peripheral compartment.

- Anterior portal
  - Many anterior portals have been described in the literature.
  - One of the most common starts at the intersection of (1) a sagittal line drawn down from the ASIS and (2) a transverse line at the superior edge of the greater trochanter.
  - Portal entry angle: start by angling the needle ~45 degrees cephalad and 30 degrees toward the midline, although the actual angle to enter the joint from the anterior portal varies significantly from patient to patient.
  - Needle passes through the rectus femoris and sartorius (should not perforate the iliopsoas tendon, which is more medial)
  - Another common anterior portal (preferred by the senior author) starts at the skin 7 cm distal and anterior/medial to the anterolateral portal.

‣ Allows for easier access to the central compartment in cases of anterior acetabular overcoverage

‣ Reduces risk of injury to the rectus femoris and the LFCN

‣ Provides better angle of approach when placing anterior acetabular anchors for labral repair/refixation

■ Allows visualization of: anterior femoral neck, anterior joint (including the anteroinferior labrum), posterior-superior joint, superior retinacular fold, and ligamentum teres

■ Protect the branches of the LFCN (on average 0.3 cm from the anterior portal) by incising the skin only and using a blunt trochar to course to the joint

■ Feel for the femoral pulse just distal to the inguinal ligament to stay away from the femoral neurovascular bundle (femoral nerve should be on average ~3.2 cm from the portal tract)

● Posterolateral/posterior paratrochanteric portal

■ Start at the superoposterior margin of the greater trochanter in line with the anterolateral portal, but approximately 1 cm posterior to the posterior superior aspect of the greater trochanter → pass through the gluteus medius and minimus muscles → angle the needle toward the tip of the camera → watch needle enter the joint through the capsule between the labrum and femoral head

■ Allows visualization of: posterior aspect of femoral head, posterior and posteroinferior labrum and capsule, inferior edge of ischiofemoral ligament, posterior ligamentum teres, lateral and anterior acetabular articular surfaces

■ At greatest risk: sciatic nerve which is on average ~2.9 cm from this portal at the level of the posterior hip capsule

‣ When establishing the portal: keep femur in neutral or slight internal rotation to rotate the nerve away from the greater trochanter posterior margin

‣ External rotation moves the greater trochanter posteriorly, reducing the margin of safety between the sciatic nerve and the portal path.

■ Superior gluteal nerve is ~4.4 cm superior to both lateral portals.

● Some surgeons using the lateral decubitus position prefer to use just the peritrochanteric portals instead.

■ Anterior superior trochanteric portal: placed at the junction of the anterior and the middle third of the superior trochanteric ridge

- Posterior superior trochanteric portal: placed at the junction of the mid and posterior third of the superior trochanteric ridge

- Both are placed as close to bone as possible, aiming cephalad parallel to femoral neck (portals are parallel).

- **Ancillary portal or accessory anterolateral (AAL) or distal anterolateral (DAL) portal**
  - 3 to 5 cm distal to the anterolateral portal along the anterior border of the greater trochanter
  - Used to access the peripheral compartment (e.g., for loose body removal, femoral head osteoplasty for cam impingement, synovectomy, addressing femoral neck lesions, iliopsoas release)

- **Mid-anterolateral portal**
  - About 2 cm distal to the midpoint of a line connecting the anterior and AL portals
  - Used for débridement of the femoral neck and anchor placement in labral repairs

- **Proximal anterolateral (PAL) portal**
  - 4 cm proximal to the anterolateral portal, in line with the shaft of the femur
  - Used for peripheral compartment access for femoral head-neck osteoplasty/cheilectomy and internal fixation of superior acetabular rim stress fracture

- **Portals for work in the peritrochanteric space (e.g., for greater trochanteric pain syndrome)** *(Fig. 3-12)*:

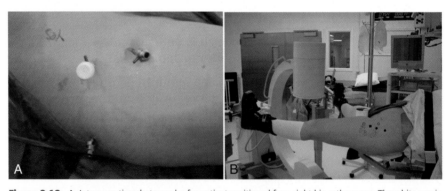

Figure 3-12. **A.** Intraoperative photograph of a patient positioned for a right hip arthroscopy. The white cap is on the anterolateral portal, while to the right and slightly medial is the modified anterior portal preferred by the senior author, and below is posterolateral portal. **B.** Shows the arthroscopy portals for peritrochanteric arthroscopy. The *open black circle* represents the peritrochanteric space portal, whereas the *black square* is the distal anterolateral accessory portal and the *complete black circle* is the proximal anterolateral accessory portal. The *open black squares* are the proximal and distal portals for trochanteric bursal surgery.

- Best access is via an anterior portal (1 cm lateral to the ASIS within the interval between the tensor fascia lata and sartorius)

  ‣ Leg position: full extension, 0 degree of adduction, 10 to 15 degrees of internal rotation

  ‣ Direct cannula posteriorly, sweep back and forth between the ITB and the greater trochanter to open up the space

- Distal posterior portal: midway between the tip of the greater trochanter and vastus tubercle along the posterior ⅓ of the greater trochanteric midline, used for distal access for operative interventions (e.g., ITB release)

- Optional third portal: proximal to the tip of the greater trochanter in line with the distal posterior portal for more proximal work and more distal visualization

Portal Placement

● Position the patient and adjust traction

  - Place the patient on the fracture table with a well-padded perineal post lateralized to the affected side (i.e., against the surgical hip medial thigh)

  - Optimal distraction vector (parallel to the femoral neck rather than the femoral shaft) decreases direct pressure on perineum/pudendal nerve

  - Make sure the groin/genitals are protected.

  - Place both feet in padded traction boots: pad the feet well and fully seat the heels in the foot-holder in neutral rotation, secure the foot and ankle well so that the heel does not lift off with traction.

  - Nonoperative leg: 45 to 60 degrees of abduction, neutral rotation, neutral flexion/extension

  - Operative leg: 10 degrees of abduction, neutral rotation

    ‣ Some surgeons prefer slight flexion of the operative leg, although the senior author prefers neutral flexion-extension.

  - Apply slight traction to the unaffected side to help lateralize the affected hip and act as a counterbalance.

  - Apply traction to the affected hip under fluoroscopic visualization.

  - Vacuum phenomenon:

    ‣ The negative intracapsular pressure that accumulates with distraction

- ‣ Seen as a crescent-shaped radiolucency on fluoroscopy

- ‣ Can release this pressure before traction: place the spinal needle into the joint under fluoroscopic visualization → creates an air arthrogram and minimizes the forces necessary to achieve adequate distraction

- ‣ Some surgeons inject saline in the joint at this point

- ‣ Otherwise the pressure is released later with spinal needle placement when establishing the first portal

  - ▪ Typically need ~20 to 50 lb of traction for distraction

- Fluoroscopic image to confirm ability to establish necessary hip distraction (look for 8–10 mm from superior femoral head to the acetabular rim)

  - ▪ Need enough distraction to decrease the risk of iatrogenic chondral injury during portal placement, intra-articular navigation, and procedures

  - ▪ Use least amount of force to achieve necessary distraction because most complications from hip arthroscopy are related to traction.

- Release traction

- Prep and drape the hip

- Reapply traction

- Spinal needle to establish the anterolateral portal with fluoroscopy as needed

  - ▪ Aim anterolaterally in the joint with the long end of the bevel of the needle away from the femoral head to avoid inadvertent articular scuffing of the femoral head.

  - ▪ Will feel a decrease in resistance as you penetrate the capsule.

  - ▪ Avoid piercing the labrum: may feel an increase in resistance if you drive into the labrum.

- Remove the stylet

- Some surgeons distend the joint with 30 to 60 mL of normal saline (may include an anesthetic) → breaks the hip suction seal, backflow of fluid confirms intra-articular placement (the senior author does not do this because the blood from the joint may obscure visualization during establishment of the second portal)

- Some surgeons remove the spinal needle, then reenter the joint after distention to decrease the incidence of labral damage.

- Stab incision on both sides of the needle

- Remove the needle over a Nitinol guidewire

- Cautiously twist a 5.0 mm cannula with blunt trochar over the wire into the joint

- Remove obturator and wire

- Insert camera with 70-degree lens through cannula
- Rotate the lens to view the interval anteriorly between the labrum and femoral head to visualize entry of the anterior spinal needle while the joint is "dry."
- Replace the spinal needle with a guidewire
- Incise the skin about the anterior guidewire, taking care not to penetrate deeply to reduce the risk of injury to the LFCN which is subcutaneous
- Place the blunt trochar with 5.0 mm cannula over the guidewire under arthroscopic visualization to ensure that the labrum and articular cartilage are protected.
- Remove the trochar
- Irrigate the joint
  - To optimize visualization: consider keeping systolic blood pressure <100 mm Hg, using dilute epinephrine in the arthroscopy fluid, radiofrequency device for coagulation as needed
- Place the camera and 70-degree lens into the anterior portal to assess whether the anterolateral portal violated the labrum. If so, reposition the cannula at this time. If not, replace the camera and lens back into the anterolateral portal.
- Establish the posterolateral portal under arthroscopic visualization in the same fashion
- Rotating the hip (by rotating the foot plate) can provide improved access to the entire joint, including the medial femoral head and the ligamentum teres.
- Maintain cannulas in position throughout the procedure to decrease risk of instrument breakage, soft tissue trauma, chondral and neurovascular damage.
- To access the hip joint peripheral compartment:
  - Remove intra-articular instruments
  - Release traction
  - Flex hip ~30 to 45 degrees (relaxes the anterior capsule)
  - Redirect the anterolateral portal onto the anterior femoral neck
  - Establish a distal anterolateral portal under direct arthroscopic visualization

Diagnostic Arthroscopy

- Each surgeon should develop a routine, systematic evaluation of the joint to be addressed before any treatment.
- Use both a 70- and 30-degree lens in all three portals to fully evaluate the entire central compartment.
- Most clinicians use a 30- or 70-degree lens to perform arthroscopy of the peripheral compartment

- Key points in the joint examination and any pathology should be imaged and kept in the patient's chart.
- Note location, size, and grade of lesions for the operative report.

Common Hip Arthroscopic Procedures

- Removal of symptomatic loose bodies: excellent results
- Labral débridement *(Fig. 3-13)*
    - Resect labrum conservatively back to a stable edge to avoid catching of the flap but avoid over-resection (especially in dysplasia)
    - Success rate ranges from 68% to 82%, less favorable results in the presence of articular damage (e.g., 21% success rate with osteoarthritis on radiographs)
    - Success rate of labral surgery in the face of untreated FAI worse than with concomitant FAI surgery

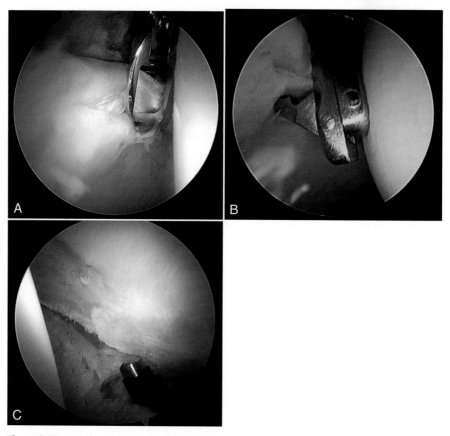

Figure 3-13. **A.** Arthroscopic photo from the anterolateral portal of a biter removing an anterior labral tear. **B.** Demonstrates a partial labrectomy being performed with a reverse biter. **C.** Arthroscopic photo from the anterolateral portal of the posterolateral labrum following radiofrequency ablation of a labral tear.

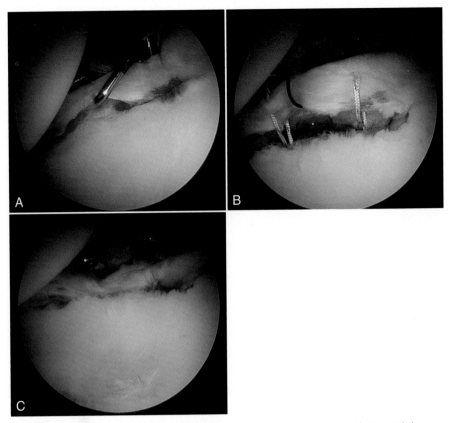

Figure 3-14. A through **C.** Scope photos of labral repair: passing suture and one with sutures tied.

- Labral repair: labrum is hypovascular, mixed results *(Fig. 3-14).*
    - Labral clefts are normal variants
    - No good studies of isolated labral repair; however, results of FAI surgery seem to be better when labral repair is performed
    - Repair usually reserved for labral-chondral separation because bleeding from bone will allow healing; repair of intrasubstance tearing has less favorable results
- Chondral lesions *(Figs. 3-15 and 3-16)*
    - Small lesions <7 mm from rim: chondroplasty alone performed
    - Large unstable flaps: excised, underlying subchondral bone is microfractured
    - Extensive lesions and bipolar lesions: poor prognosis
- Débridement of a ruptured ligamentum teres: great results, average 43 point improvement in the 100-point modified Harris hip scale at minimum 1-year follow-up

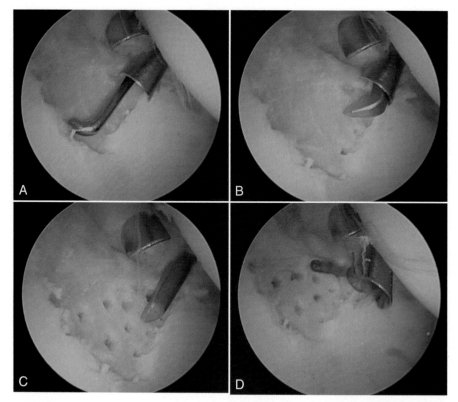

Figure 3-15. A. Arthroscopic view from the posterolateral portal of an acetabular chondral lesion in a 24-year-old woman with hip impingement and chondral injury to the anterolateral acetabulum measuring more than 1 cm from the acetabular rim. **B.** Shows the microfracture of the acetabulum in this patient. **C.** Fat being released from the microfracture holes. **D.** Demonstrates bleeding from the microfracture perforations.

- Biopsy
  - Patients who present with monoarticular inflammatory arthritis of the hip can have a hip arthroscopy to obtain a synovial biopsy for histopathologic diagnosis (to target therapy) and the surgeon can simultaneously acquire information about the extent of the synovitis and state of the articular cartilage.
- Partial synovectomy/debulking: impossible to do a complete synovectomy arthroscopically
  - Complete synovectomy requires dislocation of the femoral head, which may increase the risk of AVN (these patients are often on high dosages of steroids)
  - Significant symptomatic improvement seen in PVNS and synovial chondromatosis with arthroscopic debulking
  - At mean follow-up of 79 months for synovial chondromatosis: 57% good or excellent outcomes; 20% had undergone a THA

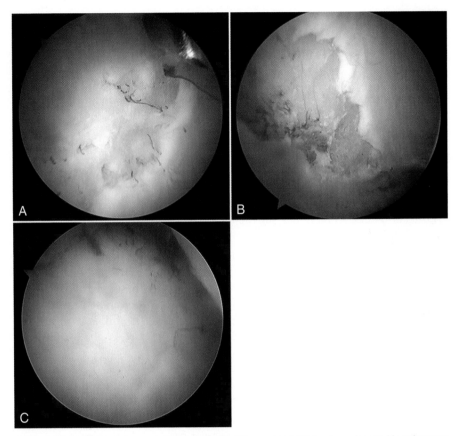

Figure 3-16. **A** and **B.** Arthroscopic photographs of a 32-year-old triathlete who underwent hip arthroscopy for femoroacetabular impingement and had an acetabular chondral lesion that was treated with chondroplasty and microfracture. **C.** A repeat arthroscopy on same patient 7 months after the microfracture demonstrating fibrocartilage growth covering 100% of the lesion.

- In a recurrent diffuse PVNS: can perform a complete synovectomy by combining arthroscopic and open techniques to avoid femoral head dislocation

- In RA: adjunct to treatment in patients in the early minimally erosive stage of the disease for symptomatic relief but also for visual assessment of the articular surface (there is often more articular damage than is apparent on radiographs) to explain intractable symptoms and to plan future treatment appropriately (e.g., THA)

- Outcomes correlate with articular cartilage integrity.

- In chondrocalcinosis: lavage, synovial debulking of the crystal-laden tissue at an early stage may slow the articular cartilage degeneration.

- Débridement of degenerative disease
  - Controversy whether débridement may be helpful for milder chondromalacia to postpone eventual THA
  - Improvement in 34% to 60% of patients
  - Consider for: younger patients with mild OA, well-preserved ROM, and realistic expectations
  - An acute change in symptoms may be a sign of a dislodged fragment that can be retrieved arthroscopically.
  - Poorer results if there is underlying FAI

- Microfracture: for grade IV lesions with well-preserved surrounding articular cartilage and intact subchondral bone (see *Figs. 3-15 and 3-16*)
  - Shaver or curette to create well-defined vertical margins, completely remove the calcified cartilage layer; maintain the integrity of the subchondral bone; use an arthroscopic awl perpendicularly to penetrate the subchondral bone with multiple holes; see marrow elements released through the holes when the water or pump pressure is lowered.
  - 86% Good results at minimum 2-year follow-up
  - On second-look arthroscopy at 10 to 36 months after the primary arthroscopy: the average percent fill of the acetabular chondral lesion was 91%.
  - Need 6 to 10 weeks of restricted weight-bearing, consider continuous passive motion (CPM) for similar amount of time to encourage fibrocartilaginous healing

- Osteoplasty for FAI *(Fig. 3-17)*
  - Outcomes similar for arthroscopic and open management of FAI
  - Hip arthroscopy may be indicated after an open procedure for adhesiolysis in those with persistent pain but no detectable osseous or cartilaginous pathology; good results if adhesions can be released
  - Central compartment arthroscopy: address labral pathology and chondral lesions; in cases of pincer impingement: removal of anterior acetabular rim and reattachment of labrum if possible
  - Peripheral compartment arthroscopy: remove cam lesions at the anterior, anterolateral, and/or lateral femoral head-neck junction ("bumpectomy" or "cheilectomy")
  - May combine arthroscopy with a limited modified open approach for decompression

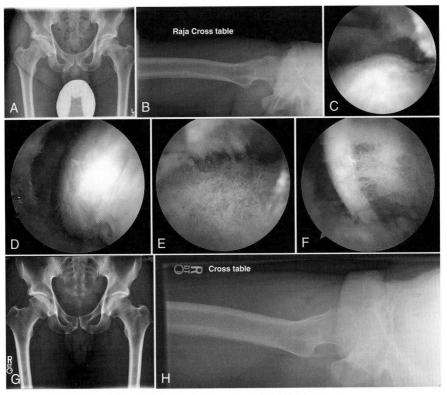

Figure 3-17. A 40-year-old male who had to give up performing martial arts due to hip pain and had increasing pain with other activities. An AP pelvis (**A**) and a lateral radiograph of the right hip (**B**), demonstrating a combined type of femoroacetabular impingement with a large cam lesion. Arthroscopic views of the cam lesion anteriorly (**C**) and laterally (**D**). **E.** Arthroscopic view of the anterofemoral head and neck junction after chielectomy/femoral osteoplasty. **F.** Demonstrates the lateral femoral head and neck junction after decompression. **G.** AP pelvis radiograph and **H.** Lateral radiograph 6 months after arthroscopic surgery for FAI in this patient.

- Excision of impinging osteophytes: successful in post-traumatic cases but less predictable results in degenerative cases because of associated joint pathology

- Significant improvement in function, pain, and ROM postoperatively

- 42 of 45 (93%) of professional athletes returned to professional competition following arthroscopic decompression of FAI (the other three had diffuse OA)

- Need long-term follow-up and studies investigating possible alterations in the natural history of OA in these patients

- Synovectomy for inflammatory arthritides (e.g., RA, synovial chondromatosis, and PVNS): need to enter the peripheral compartment for a complete synovectomy and for loose body removal

- Capsulorrhaphy for symptomatic instability (e.g., Ehlers-Danlos syndrome)

  - Thermal capsular shrinkage versus suture plication

  - Thermal energy → inflammatory cascade in the capsule → fibroplastic response → secondary capsular thickening

    ‣ Average improvement of 38 points in the 100-point modified Harris hip scale at 2- to 5-year follow-up in a cohort of four hips

  - Jargon may be better in the hip versus the shoulder due to the much thicker capsule and more inherent bony stability.

  - Suture plication of the iliofemoral ligament also found to be successful, but more difficult to perform compared with jargon capsulorrhaphy

  - Anecdotal reports suggest that both are beneficial.

  - Difficult to study due to lack of validated outcomes measure and lack of objective measurement of laxity/instability

- Irrigation and débridement of an acute septic hip
- Manipulation under anesthesia with concomitant arthroscopy for adhesive capsulitis: see characteristic capsular fibrosis with hemorrhagic fibrinous debris on arthroscopy, very effective treatment, especially if there is no radiographic evidence of OA
- Occasionally arthroscopic lysis of adhesions (particularly following labral repair) when the capsule adheres to the labrum, limiting motion
- Arthroscopic reduction and internal fixation of osteochondral fractures of the acetabulum (using percutaneous lag screws) *(Fig. 3-18)* and of the femoral head (using a Herbert screw)
- Release of a snapping hip:

  - Internal snapping hip: iliopsoas lengthening *(Fig. 3-19)*

    ‣ From within the central compartment: identify tendon through a small window in the anterior capsule, transect through a 1-cm medial capsular window adjacent to the anterior portal.

    ‣ From within the peripheral compartment: in 20% the tendon is seen within the peripheral compartment; otherwise, a 1-cm transverse capsulotomy is made just lateral to the medial synovial fold (just proximal to the zona orbicularis).

    ‣ Release at its insertion on the lesser trochanter:

      • Position the hip in 15 degrees of flexion and external rotation

      • Make a distal anterolateral portal and another portal 3 cm distal to that

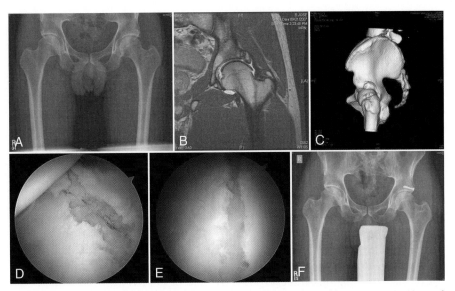

Figure 3-18. An AP pelvis radiograph (**A**) of a 32-year-old triathlete with hip impingement and evidence of an acetabular roof stress fracture, confirmed on MRI (**B**) demonstrating that the fragment, if removed, would result in iatrogenic dysplasia of the hip. A 3D CT scan (**C**) also clearly shows the fracture fragment. **D.** Arthroscopic view of the stress fracture after débridement of the fibrous tissue from the non-union site. **E,.** Arthroscopic view following arthroscopic débridement, reduction, and internal fixation of the fragment, demonstrating excellent reduction and that the articular surface is not violated by the screws. **F.** Radiograph postoperatively of the patient with the internal fixation of the stress fracture fragment that healed uneventfully and allowed full return to competition by this triathlete.

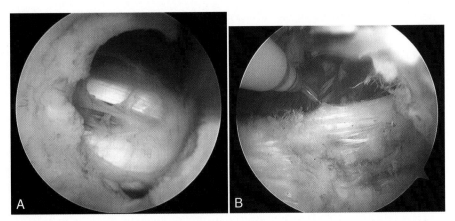

Figure 3-19. A. Arthroscopic view in the peripheral compartment after making a capsulotomy revealing the iliopsoas tendon. **B.** Endoscopic view of an electrocautery at the iliopsoas tendon at its insertion onto the lesser trochanter.

- Bring the trochar/cannula from the distal portal and a shaver from the proximal portal to the lesser trochanter under fluoroscopic visualization

- Clear out the iliopsoas bursa just proximal to the lesser trochanter to help expose the iliopsoas tendon

- Anecdotal reports of increased risk of HO when using this approach

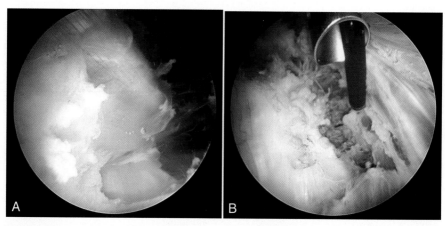

Figure 3-20. A and **B.** Photographs of an arthroscopic iliotibial band partial resection for coxa saltans externa.

- External snapping hip: release posterior third of the ITB over the greater trochanter from the ITB undersurface through a proximal lateral accessory portal (*Fig. 3-20*)
  - Alternatively, portals can be made 4 cm proximal and distal to the apex of the lateral aspect of the greater trochanter.
    ▸ Clear the soft tissue over the ITB.
  - Using a radiofrequency device, a cruciate or bicruciate incision may be made in the ITB over the greater trochanter.
    ▸ The free edges may be resected, leaving an oval defect in the ITB, as is done with the open technique.
  - Occasionally the gluteus maximus tendon is the culprit (can be released arthroscopically from the linea aspira).
- Trochanteric bursectomy: make portals 4 cm proximal and distal to the apex of the lateral aspect of the trochanter, clear the soft tissue over the ITB, incise the ITB along its posterior border, excise the bursa over the greater trochanter using a shaver and/or a radiofrequency probe brought under the ITB.
- Hip abductor repair: may be performed by entering the peritrochanteric space under the ITB. The gluteus medius and/or minimus tendons may be repaired to the greater trochanter using suture anchors and arthroscopic suture-passing devices, similar to an arthroscopic rotator cuff repair.

Prognosis

- In general, outcomes are highly dependent on the degree of articular cartilage pathology; arthritis is an indicator of poor short- and long-term outcomes.

- 10-Year follow-up study

  - Greatest improvement seen in first month; at 3 months, improvement begins to plateau; still gradual improvement for the first year; at 2 years: improvement maintained; at 5 years: improvement diminished slightly; at 10 years: results approach the 2-year level

  - Best results: removal of symptomatic loose bodies

  - Good sustained results for treatment of synovial disease and labral and chondral lesions in the absence of degenerative disease

- For FAI surgery with intact articular cartilage: patients have 80% of the improvement in the first 6 months, 95% by 1 year.

Revision Hip Arthroscopy

- Patients requiring revision arthroscopy typically present with groin pain that is worse with activity, no significant improvement with conservative measures. and decreased ROM on examination.

- 60% to 79% of revision arthroscopy patients had FAI bony lesions addressed at the time of revision that had not been addressed (or had been inadequately addressed) at the index procedure.

  - In patients with evidence of FAI on radiographs, there is a significantly higher proportion of patients with excellent/good results in the osteoplasty with labral débridement group as compared to the group with only labral débridement.

Postoperative Care

- May inject an anesthetic (e.g., ropivacaine) into the joint at the completion of the procedure. Avoid steroids because they may increase the risk of infection.

- Leave hospital on day of surgery.

- Narcotic medications and stool softeners postoperatively

- NSAIDs for 3 weeks postoperatively for DVT and HO prophylaxis when concomitant bony procedures (e.g., cheilectomy and/or acetabuloplasty) or an iliopsoas release are performed

- Formal DVT prophylaxis for those with history of DVT or distance travel in first 6 weeks postoperatively

- Place patient in hip brace if labrum repaired (avoids hyperflexion and external rotation) for first 10 to 14 days postoperatively (Fig. 3-21)

- Weight-bearing as tolerated with crutches for hip arthroscopy except if labral repair, cheilectomy, or microfracture was performed

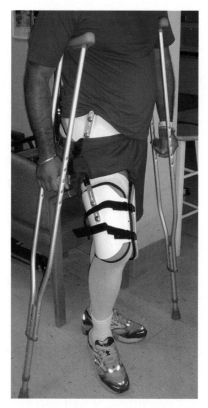

Figure 3-21. Photograph of a patient with a hip abduction brace used to limit hip flexion and abduction.

- Foot flat partial weight-bearing (20 lb) with crutches for 2 weeks if labral repair and/or osteoplasty/cheilectomy for men <60 and women <40 years; add an extra week of limited weight-bearing postoperatively for every decade beyond these ages
- Continuous passive motion (CPM) for 6 hours per day for 2 weeks for most hip arthroscopy; 8 hours per day for 8 weeks if microfracture performed
- Passive hip circumduction exercises with hip at 70 degrees of flexion for first 2 weeks postoperatively to reduce risk of adhesions
- Cold therapy with compression may be beneficial postoperatively for pain relief and early transition from narcotics
- Sutures out ~postoperative day 10 to 14
- Postoperative physical therapy for 3 to 6 months
- Rehabilitation goals: control swelling and pain to minimize muscle inhibition and atrophy; early ROM and initiation of muscle activity and neuromuscular control; progressive lower extremity resisted exercises
- Resume sport-specific activities by the 4th month except if microfracture (running is postponed for 6 months in these cases)

Complications

- Rates range from 0.5% to 6.4%
- Most common complications: transient neurapraxias of the pudendal, LFCN, sciatic, peroneal, and femoral nerves
  - Best to keep traction as brief as possible (<2 hours is optimal) and only as much force as needed to distract the joint sufficiently (although duration of traction is a greater risk factor than amount of traction)
  - Neurologic symptoms usually subside within 6 to 8 weeks.
  - Other traction-related complications: damage to knee and ankle ligaments, pressure necrosis of the foot, scrotum, or perineum
- Iatrogenic chondral scuffing and labral perforation (particularly on entry into the joint): probably the most common complication but is largely under-reported
- Direct trauma to neurovascular structures
  - Greatest risk of nerve injury with portal placement is to LFCN when establishing the anterior portal, causes reduced sensation in the lateral thigh, incidence ~ 0.5%, minimize risk by placing portal 1 cm lateral to the ASIS and by incising only the skin
  - Catastrophic: direct injury to sciatic nerve or femoral neurovascular structures
- Fluid extravasation into the retroperitoneal and intraperitoneal cavities: suspect if sudden drop in body temperature and/or blood pressure with abdominal swelling and discomfort
  - Potentially fatal: may lead to abdominal compartment syndrome or cardiac arrest
  - Associated with recent acetabular fractures, extra-articular procedures, and prolonged surgical times with use of arthroscopic pump irrigation
  - May require paracentesis or emergent laparotomy to relieve excessive intra-abdominal pressure
- Incomplete reshaping of FAI deformity, potentially necessitating revision surgery
- Trochanteric bursitis
- Hemarthrosis
- Instrument breakage
- Infection
- Femoral neck fracture after arthroscopic cam remodeling

- In cadaveric study: resection of up to 30% of the femoral head-neck junction anterolateral quadrant did not affect the proximal femur load-bearing capacity; >30% resection → 20% decrease in energy required to produce a fracture

- Hip subluxation/dislocation: may result from excessive labral débridement or bone removal from the acetabular rim in patients with hip dysplasia
- Recommend no bone resection in cases with center-edge angles of 20 degrees or less
- Femoral head AVN (very rare)
- Anesthesia complications
- DVT/pulmonary embolism (PE): only case of a fatal PE after a hip arthroscopy was reported in a polytraumatized patient, currently no guidelines for DVT prophylaxis after hip arthroscopy
- Reflex sympathetic dystrophy/complex regional pain syndrome
- Instrument failure: remove broken pieces if an instrument breaks
- Intra-articular adhesions/painful joint stiffness

REFERENCES

Awan N and Murray P. Role of hip arthroscopy in the diagnosis and treatment of hip joint pathology. *Arthroscopy* 2006; 22:215–218.

Bardakos NV, Vasconcelos JC, and Villar RN. Early outcome of hip arthroscopy for femoroacetabular impingement: The role of femoral osteoplasty in symptomatic improvement. *J Bone Joint Surg Br* 2008; 90:1570–1575.

Bartlett CS, DiFelice GS, Buly RL, et al. Cardiac arrest as a result of intraabdominal extravasation of fluid during arthroscopic removal of a loose body from the hip joint of a patient with an acetabular fracture. *J Orthop Trauma* 1998; 12:294–299.

Beaule PE, O'Neill M, and Rakhra K. Acetabular labral tears. *J Bone Joint Surg Am* 2009; 91:701–710.

Beaule PE, Clohisy JC, Schoenecker P, et al. Hip arthroscopy: An emerging gold standard. *Arthroscopy* 2007; 23:682.

Benali Y and Katthagen BD. Hip subluxation as a complication of arthroscopic débridement. *Arthroscopy* 2009; 25:405–407.

Berend KR and Vail TP. Hip arthroscopy in the adolescent and pediatric athlete. *Clin Sports Med* 2001; 20:763–778.

Bharam S. Labral tears, extra-articular injuries, and hip arthroscopy in the athlete. *Clin Sports Med* 2006; 25:279–292.

Biant LC, Bruce WJ, van der Wall H, and Walsh WR. Infection or allergy in the painful metal-on-metal total hip arthroplasty? *J Arthroplasty* 2010 Feb; 25(2):334.

Bond JL, Knutson ZA, Ebert A, and Guanche CA. The 23-point arthroscopic examination of the hip: Basic setup, portal placement, and surgical technique. *Arthroscopy* 2009; 25:416–429.

Bonnomet F, Clavert P, Abidine FZ, et al. Hip arthroscopy in hereditary multiple exostoses: A new perspective of treatment. *Arthroscopy* 2001; 17:E40.

Boyer T and Dorfmann H. Arthroscopy in primary synovial chondromatosis of the hip: Description and outcome of treatment. *J Bone Joint Surg Br* 2008; 90:314–318.

Brunner A, Horisberger M, and Herzog RF. Sports and recreation activity of patients with femoroacetabular impingement before and after arthroscopic osteoplasty. *Am J Sports Med* 2009; 37:917–922.

Burman MS. Arthroscopy or the direct visualization of joints: An experimental cadaver study. 1931. *Clin Orthop Relat Res* 2001; (390):5–9.

Burnett RS, Della Rocca GJ, Prather H, et al. Clinical presentation of patients with tears of the acetabular labrum. *J Bone Joint Surg Am* 2006; 88:1448–1457.

Bushnell BD and Dahners LE. Fatal pulmonary embolism in a polytraumatized patient following hip arthroscopy. *Orthopedics* 2009; 32:56.

Byrd JW. Hip arthroscopy. *J Am Acad Orthop Surg* 2006; 14:433–444.

Byrd JW. The role of hip arthroscopy in the athletic hip. *Clin Sports Med* 2006; 25:255–278, viii.

Byrd JW. Hip arthroscopy: Surgical indications. *Arthroscopy* 2006; 22:1260–1262.

Byrd JW and Jones KS. Hip arthroscopy for labral pathology: Prospective analysis with 10-year follow-up. *Arthroscopy* 2009; 25:365–368.

Byrd JW and Jones KS. Prospective analysis of hip arthroscopy with 10-year followup. *Clin Orthop Relat Res* 2010; 468(3):741–746.

Byrd JW and Jones KS. Adhesive capsulitis of the hip. *Arthroscopy* 2006; 22:89–94.

Byrd JW and Jones KS. Traumatic rupture of the ligamentum teres as a source of hip pain. *Arthroscopy* 2004; 20:385–391.

Byrd JW and Jones KS. Hip arthroscopy in the presence of dysplasia. *Arthroscopy* 2003; 19:1055–1060.

Byrd JW. Hip arthroscopy. The supine position. *Clin Sports Med* 2001; 20:703–731.

Byrd JW and Jones KS. Hip arthroscopy in athletes. *Clin Sports Med* 2001; 20:749–761.

Byrd JW. Avoiding the labrum in hip arthroscopy. *Arthroscopy* 2000; 16:770–773.

Byrd JW, Pappas JN, and Pedley MJ. Hip arthroscopy: An anatomic study of portal placement and relationship to the extra-articular structures. *Arthroscopy* 1995; 11:418–423.

Clarke MT, Arora A, and Villar RN. Hip arthroscopy: Complications in 1054 cases. *Clin Orthop Relat Res* 2003; (406):84–88.

Clohisy JC and McClure JT. Treatment of anterior femoroacetabular impingement with combined hip arthroscopy and limited anterior decompression. *Iowa Orthop J* 2005; 25:164–171.

Cory JW and Ruch DS. Arthroscopic removal of a 44 caliber bullet from the hip. *Arthroscopy* 1998; 14:624–626.

Crnobaric A, Blagojevic Z, and Stevanovic V. Arthroscopy of the hip—surgical treatment of synovial osteochondromatosis. *Acta Chir Iugosl* 2006; 53:121–123.

DeAngelis NA and Busconi BD. Hip arthroscopy in the pediatric population. *Clin Orthop Relat Res* 2003; 406:60–63.

DeAngelis NA and Busconi BD. Assessment and differential diagnosis of the painful hip. *Clin Orthop Relat Res* 2003; 406:11–18.

Dienst M and Kohn D. Arthroscopic treatment of femoroacetabular impingement technique and results. *Orthopade* 2009; 38:429–443.

Dienst M, Godde S, Seil R, et al. Hip arthroscopy without traction: In vivo anatomy of the peripheral hip joint cavity. *Arthroscopy* 2001; 17:924–931.

Diulus CA, Krebs VE, Hanna G, and Barsoum WK. Hip arthroscopy technique and indications. *J Arthroplasty* 2006; 21:68–73.

Dorfmann H and Boyer T. Arthroscopy of the hip: 12 years of experience. *Arthroscopy* 1999; 15:67–72.

Edwards DJ, Lomas D, and Villar RN. Diagnosis of the painful hip by magnetic resonance imaging and arthroscopy. *J Bone Joint Surg Br* 1995; 77:374–376.

Farjo LA, Glick JM, and Sampson TG. Hip arthroscopy for acetabular labral tears. *Arthroscopy* 1999; 15:137.

Friend L and Kelly BT. Femoroacetabular impingement and labral tears in the adolescent hip: Diagnosis and surgical advances. *Curr Opin Pediatr* 2009; 21:71–76.

Glick JM. Hip arthroscopy. The lateral approach. *Clin Sports Med* 2001; 20:733–747.

Gokhale S, Khan M, Kuiper JH, et al. An arthroscopic hip documentation form. *Arthroscopy* 2008; 24:839–842.

Griffin KM. Rehabilitation of the hip. *Clin Sports Med* 2001; 20:837–850, viii.

Hamilton LC, Biant LC, Temple LN, and Field RE. Isolated pseudogout diagnosed on hip arthroscopy. *J Bone Joint Surg Br* 2009; 91:533–535.

Haupt U, Volkle D, Waldherr C, and Beck M. Intra- and retroperitoneal irrigation liquid after arthroscopy of the hip joint. *Arthroscopy* 2008; 24:966–968.

Heyworth BE, Shindle MK, Voos JE, et al. Radiologic and intraoperative findings in revision hip arthroscopy. *Arthroscopy* 2007; 23:1295–1302.

Ilizaliturri Jr VM. Complications of arthroscopic femoroacetabular impingement treatment: A review. *Clin Orthop Relat Res* 2009; 467:760–768.

Ilizaliturri Jr VM, Byrd JW, Sampson TG, et al. A geographic zone method to describe intra-articular pathology in hip arthroscopy: Cadaveric study and preliminary report. *Arthroscopy* 2008; 24:534–539.

Ilizaliturri Jr VM, Acosta-Rodriguez E, and Camacho-Galindo J. A minimalist approach to hip arthroscopy: The slotted cannula. *Arthroscopy* 2007; 23:560.e1–e3.

Ilizaliturri Jr VM, Zarate-Kalfopulos B, Martinez-Escalante FA, et al. Arthroscopic retrieval of a broken guidewire fragment from the hip joint after cannulated screw fixation of slipped capital femoral epiphysis. *Arthroscopy* 2007; 23:227.e1–e4.

Kamath AF, Componovo R, Baldwin K, et al. Hip arthroscopy for labral tears: Review of clinical outcomes with 4.8-year mean follow-up. *Am J Sports Med* 2009; 37(9):1721–1727.

Kelly BT and Buly RL. Hip arthroscopy update. *HSS J* 2005; 1:40–48.

Kelly BT, Weiland DE, Schenker ML, and Philippon MJ. Arthroscopic labral repair in the hip: Surgical technique and review of the literature. *Arthroscopy* 2005; 21:1496–1504.

Kelly BT, Williams RJ 3rd, and Philippon MJ. Hip arthroscopy: Current indications, treatment options, and management issues. *Am J Sports Med* 2003; 31:1020–1037.

Khanduja V and Villar RN. The role of arthroscopy in resurfacing arthroplasty of the hip. *Arthroscopy* 2008; 24:122.e1–e3.

Kim KC, Hwang DS, Lee CH, and Kwon ST. Influence of femoroacetabular impingement on results of hip arthroscopy in patients with early osteoarthritis. *Clin Orthop Relat Res* 2007; 456:128–132.

Kim SJ, Choi NH, and Kim HJ. Operative hip arthroscopy. *Clin Orthop Relat Res* 1998; (353):156–165.

Kocher MS and Tucker R. Pediatric athlete hip disorders. *Clin Sports Med* 2006; 25:241–253, viii.

Kocher MS, Kim YJ, Millis MB, et al. Hip arthroscopy in children and adolescents. *J Pediatr Orthop* 2005; 25:680–686.

Krebs VE. The role of hip arthroscopy in the treatment of synovial disorders and loose bodies. *Clin Orthop Relat Res* 2003; (406):48–59.

Krueger A, Leunig M, Siebenrock KA, and Beck M. Hip arthroscopy after previous surgical hip dislocation for femoroacetabular impingement. *Arthroscopy* 2007; 23:1285–1289.

Larson CM and Giveans MR. Arthroscopic management of femoroacetabular impingement: Early outcomes measures. *Arthroscopy* 2008; 24:540–546.

Larson CM, Swaringen J, and Morrison G. A review of hip arthroscopy and its role in the management of adult hip pain. *Iowa Orthop J* 2005; 25:172–179.

Lincoln M, Johnston K, Muldoon M, and Santore R. Combined arthroscopic and modified open approach for cam femoroacetabular impingement: A preliminary experience. *Arthroscopy* 2009; 25:392–399.

Lo YP, Chan YS, Lien LC, et al. Complications of hip arthroscopy: Analysis of seventy three cases. *Chang Gung Med J* 2006; 29:86–92.

Lu KH. Arthroscopically assisted replacement of dynamic hip screw for unrecognized joint penetration of lag screw through a new portal. *Arthroscopy* 2004; 20:201–205.

Lubowitz JH and Poehling GG. Hip arthroscopy: An emerging gold standard. *Arthroscopy* 2006; 22:1257–1259.

Mason JB, McCarthy JC, O'Donnell J, et al. Hip arthroscopy: Surgical approach, positioning, and distraction. *Clin Orthop Relat Res* 2003; 406:29–37.

Matsuda DK. A rare fracture, an even rarer treatment: The arthroscopic reduction and internal fixation of an isolated femoral head fracture. *Arthroscopy* 2009; 25:408–412.

McCarthy J, Barsoum W, Puri L, Lee JA, Murphy S, and Cooke P. The role of hip arthroscopy in the elite athlete. *Clin Orthop Relat Res* 2003; 406:71–74.

McCarthy J, Puri L, Barsoum W, et al. Articular cartilage changes in avascular necrosis: An arthroscopic evaluation. *Clin Orthop Relat Res* 2003; 406:64–70.

McCarthy JC. Hip arthroscopy: Applications and technique. *J Am Acad Orthop Surg* 1995; 3:115–122.

McCarthy JC, Jibodh SR, and Lee JA. The role of arthroscopy in evaluation of painful hip arthroplasty. *Clin Orthop Relat Res* 2009; 467:174–180.

McCarthy JC and Lee J. Hip arthroscopy: Indications and technical pearls. *Clin Orthop Relat Res* 2005; 441:180–187.

McCarthy JC and Lee JA. Arthroscopic intervention in early hip disease. *Clin Orthop Relat Res* 2004; 429:157–162.

Meyer NJ, Thiel B, and Ninomiya JT. Retrieval of an intact, intraarticular bullet by hip arthroscopy using the lateral approach. *J Orthop Trauma* 2002; 16:51–53.

Monahan E and Shimada K. Verifying the effectiveness of a computer-aided navigation system for arthroscopic hip surgery. *Stud Health Technol Inform* 2008; 132:302–307.

Mullis BH and Dahners LE. Hip arthroscopy to remove loose bodies after traumatic dislocation. *J Orthop Trauma* 2006; 20:22–26.

Murphy KP, Ross AE, Javernick MA, and Lehman RA Jr, Repair of the adult acetabular labrum. *Arthroscopy* 2006; 22:567.e1–e3.

Nepple JJ, Zebala LP, and Clohisy JC. Labral disease associated with femoroacetabular impingement: Do we need to correct the structural deformity? *J Arthroplasty* 2009 Sep; 24(6 Suppl):114–119.

O'leary JA, Berend K, and Vail TP. The relationship between diagnosis and outcome in arthroscopy of the hip. *Arthroscopy* 2001; 17:181–188.

Pardiwala DN and Nagda TV. Arthroscopic chondral cyst excision in a stiff Perthes' hip. *Arthroscopy* 2007; 23:909.e1–e4.

Parvizi J, Bican O, Bender B, et al. Arthroscopy for labral tears in patients with developmental dysplasia of the hip: A cautionary note. *J Arthroplasty* 2009; 24(Suppl):110–113.

Philippon MJ, Briggs KK, Yen YM, and Kuppersmith DA. Outcomes following hip arthroscopy for femoroacetabular impingement with associated chondrolabral dysfunction: Minimum two-year follow-up. *J Bone Joint Surg Br* 2009; 91:16–23.

Philippon MJ, Kuppersmith DA, Wolff AB, and Briggs KK. Arthroscopic findings following traumatic hip dislocation in 14 professional athletes. *Arthroscopy* 2009; 25:169–174.

Philippon MJ, Schenker ML, Briggs KK, and Maxwell RB. Can microfracture produce repair tissue in acetabular chondral defects? *Arthroscopy* 2008; 24:46–50.

Philippon MJ, Yen YM, Briggs KK, et al. Early outcomes after hip arthroscopy for femoroacetabular impingement in the athletic adolescent patient: A preliminary report. *J Pediatr Orthop* 2008; 28:705–710.

Philippon MJ, Schenker ML, Briggs KK, et al. Revision hip arthroscopy. *Am J Sports Med* 2007; 35:1918–1921.

Robertson WJ and Kelly BT. The safe zone for hip arthroscopy: A cadaveric assessment of central, peripheral, and lateral compartment portal placement. *Arthroscopy* 2008; 24:1019–1026.

Sampson TG. Complications of hip arthroscopy. *Techniques in Orthopaedics* 2005; 20:63–66.

Santori N and Villar RN. Acetabular labral tears: Result of arthroscopic partial limbectomy. *Arthroscopy* 2000; 16:11–15.

Sharma A, Sachdev H, and Gomillion M. Abdominal compartment syndrome during hip arthroscopy. *Anaesthesia* 2009; 64:567–569.

Shetty VD and Shetty GM. Arthroscopic view of transient synovitis of the hip joint: A case report. *Knee Surg Sports Traumatol Arthrosc* 2009; 17:1003–1005.

Shetty VD and Villar RN. Hip arthroscopy: Current concepts and review of literature. *Br J Sports Med* 2007; 41:64–68; discussion 68.

Shindle MK, Voos JE, Heyworth BE, et al. Hip arthroscopy in the athletic patient: Current techniques and spectrum of disease. *J Bone Joint Surg Am* 2007; 89 (Suppl 3):29–43.

Sierra RJ, Trousdale RT, Ganz R, and Leunig M. Hip disease in the young, active patient: Evaluation and nonarthroplasty surgical options. *J Am Acad Orthop Surg* 2008; 16:689–703.

Singh PJ, Constable L, and O'Donnell J. Arthroscopic excision of a giant-cell tumour of the ligamentum teres. *J Bone Joint Surg Br* 2009; 91:809–811.

Singleton SB, Joshi A, Schwartz MA, and Collinge CA. Arthroscopic bullet removal from the acetabulum. *Arthroscopy* 2005; 21:360–364.

Smart LR, Oetgen M, Noonan B, and Medvecky M. Beginning hip arthroscopy: Indications, positioning, portals, basic techniques, and complications. *Arthroscopy* 2007; 23:1348–1353.

Sozen YV, Ozkan K, Goksan SB, et al. Arthroscopic diagnosis and treatment of an acetabular labrum bucket handle tear: A case report. *Arch Orthop Trauma Surg* 2005; 125:649–652.

Streich NA, Gotterbarm T, Barie A, and Schmitt H. Prognostic value of chondral defects on the outcome after arthroscopic treatment of acetabular labral tears. *Knee Surg Sports Traumatol Arthrosc* 2009; 17(10):1257–1263.

Svoboda SJ, Williams DM, and Murphy KP. Hip arthroscopy for osteochondral loose body removal after a posterior hip dislocation. *Arthroscopy* 2003; 19:777–781.

Sweeney HJ. Arthroscopy of the hip. Anatomy and portals. *Clin Sports Med* 2001; 20:697–702.

Takagi K. The arthroscope: The second report. *J Orthop Sci* 1939; 14:441–466.

Takagi K. The classic. arthroscope. J. Jap. Orthop. Assoc., 1939. *Clin Orthop Relat Res* 1982; (167):6–8.

Teloken MA, Schmietd I, and Tomlinson DP. Hip arthroscopy: A unique infero-medial approach to bullet removal. *Arthroscopy* 2002; 18:E21.

Tibor LM and Sekiya JK. Differential diagnosis of pain around the hip joint. *Arthroscopy* 2008; 24:1407–1421.

Verhelst L, De Schepper J, Sergeant G, et al. Variations in serum electrolyte concentrations and renal function after therapeutic hip arthroscopy: A pilot study. *Arthroscopy* 2009; 25:377–381.

Voos JE, Rudzki JR, Shindle MK, et al. Arthroscopic anatomy and surgical techniques for peritrochanteric space disorders in the hip. *Arthroscopy* 2007; 23:1246. e1–e5.

Walton NP, Jahromi I, and Lewis PL. Chondral degeneration and therapeutic hip arthroscopy. *Int Orthop* 2004; 28:354–356.

Yusaf MA and Hame SL. Arthroscopy of the hip. *Curr Sports Med Rep* 2008; 7:269–274.

Zumstein M, Hahn F, Sukthankar A, et al. How accurately can the acetabular rim be trimmed in hip arthroscopy for pincer-type femoral acetabular impingement: A cadaveric investigation. *Arthroscopy* 2009; 25:164–168.

CHAPTER 4

ANKLE ARTHROSCOPY

Zackary D. Vaughn, Kenneth J. Hunt,
and Marc R. Safran

Introduction

- Ankle joint was initially thought to be anatomically too restrictive for arthroscopy (Burman, 1931).
- Advances in the field of arthroscopy from Japanese surgeons (Takagi and Watanabe) led to more widespread use and application to ankle joint in the 1970s.
- Watanabe published his series of 28 ankle arthroscopies in 1972.
- Numerous published studies and advances over last 40 years
- Developed into key modality for treatment of post-traumatic injuries and other acute and chronic disorders
- Limited role in diagnosis only (only 26% to 43% success of ankle arthroscopy in absence of preoperative diagnosis)
- Can be utilized for treatment of both anterior and posterior pathology
- Expansion to periarticular problems, particularly tendoscopy of the peroneal, posterior tibial, and FHL tendon sheaths
- Performed much less frequently than arthroscopy of the knee or shoulder
- Complication rate is higher than knee or shoulder arthroscopy

Preoperative Considerations

▶ History and Physical Examination

- Know all relevant history including injury patterns, prior treatments and the success or failure of each, progression and characterization of symptoms. Perform a thorough examination and review all relevant imaging.
- Location of pain may provide clue to diagnosis or differential diagnosis
- Assess range of motion of the tibiotalar and subtalar joints, location of tenderness, swelling deformity, strength testing in all planes, gait (heel to toe, toe to toe, heel to heel), alignment of the hindfoot and forefoot, laxity of the tibiotalar and subtalar joint. Complete motor and sensory evaluation.
- Imaging
  - Plain radiographs of the ankle
    - ▸ AP, lateral, mortise views

   ▸ May reveal osteochondral lesions, arthritis, distal tibial and talar osteophytes, calcifications, loose bodies, syndesmosis injuries and fractures

   ■ Stress radiographs

   ▸ Anterior drawer and talar tilt tests

   ▸ May reveal tibiotalar or subtalar instability, and rotational stress testing may demonstrate injury to the syndesmosis.

   ■ MRI

   ▸ May demonstrate soft tissue sources of pain and effusion including ligament injuries, tendon injuries, impinging scar tissue, loose bodies and integrity of the overlying articular cartilage in osteochondral injuries.

● A diagnostic intra-articular injection may be useful preoperatively to help determine if the source of the pain is intra-articular to verify the utility of arthroscopy.

Indications

● Diagnostic indications include unexplained pain, swelling, locking, catching, stiffness, hemarthrosis, evaluation of syndesmosis stability and ligament injuries.

● Therapeutic indications include

   ■ Treatment of injuries to articular cartilage (i.e., chondral and osteochondral lesions)

   ■ Anterior ankle impingement

   ■ Synovectomy

   ■ Loose body removal

   ■ Reduction and fixation of some ankle fractures

   ■ Irrigation for septic joints

   ■ Arthrofibrosis

   ■ Biopsy

   ■ Assistance in fracture fixation, arthrodesis and ankle ligament reconstruction procedures.

● Contraindications include moderate-to-severe arthritis and limited motion, significantly reduced joint space, vascular compromise, complex regional pain syndrome, significant edema and local soft tissue or intra-articular infection.

Positioning

- Classically the patient is positioned supine, although many techniques have been described including the lateral position and a prone position for arthroscopy of the posterior hindfoot.
- In the supine position, the operative leg is allowed to flex at the knee and hang over the break in the table with the foot of the table lowered to allow for relaxation of the gastrocnemius complex
- Various distraction techniques can be used and are recommended.
  - Commercially available sterile distraction straps are available for noninvasive distraction *(Fig. 4-1A,B).*
  - Invasive distraction techniques have been described with variations of the external fixator; however, this is less common.
  - A loop of sterile gauze roll may also be used with manual distraction with the surgeon's foot pulling a loop to the floor.
- Posterior ankle arthroscopy is performed prone and often without distraction.

Equipment

- A standard 4.0-mm, 30-degree arthroscope may be used (and preferred by the senior author), although a smaller 2.7-mm arthroscope may be helpful and is available in a shorter version to reduce the lever arm
- A traction device (noninvasive or invasive/external distractor) is used.
- A tourniquet may be used, and is based on surgeon preference.
- Gravity inflow is often adequate; however, an arthroscopic pump can be used with caution.
- Small joint arthroscopic equipment should be available

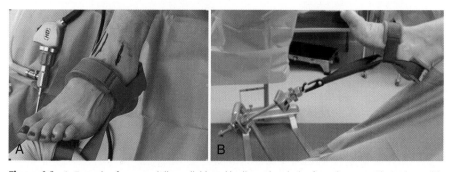

Figure 4-1. **A.** Example of commercially available ankle distraction device for arthroscopy. Shown here with knee flexed over break in table with weights applied for distraction. **B.** Ankle distraction device with knee flexed over padded leg holder with traction apparatus attached to table for distraction. Lowering the foot of the bed can result in additional distraction.

- Standard size and small joint (2.0 mm and 2.7 mm) shavers and high speed burrs, pituitary rongeurs, small joint arthroscopic graspers, rasps, and probes, miniset probes and biters, microfracture picks, cup and ring curettes

- A 70-degree arthroscope may also be helpful to visualize the medial and lateral gutters and the posterior ankle joint.

Relevant Anatomy

- An understanding of the superficial and intra-articular anatomy is key to avoiding complications from ankle arthroscopy *(Fig. 4-2A,B).*

- The neurovascular structures and tendons are at greatest risk with portal placement.

- The medial and lateral malleoli are key palpable landmarks and are useful for identifying the joint line because this typically is felt with dorsiflexion and plantar flexion of the ankle and is located approximately 2 cm proximal to the tip of the fibula and 1 cm proximal to the tip of the medial malleolus.

- Key structures to identify before portal placement that can be traced with a marking pen include the palpable dorsalis pedis artery, tibialis anterior and

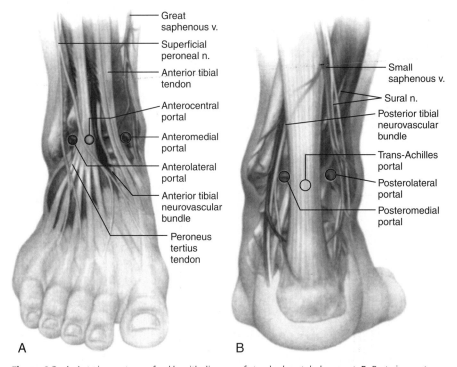

Figure 4-2. A. Anterior anatomy of ankle with diagram of standard portal placement. **B.** Posterior anatomy of ankle with diagram of standard portal placement. *(From Ferkel RD, Heath DD, Guhl JF. Neurological complications of ankle arthroscopy. Arthroscopy 1996; 12(2):200-208.)*

peroneus tertius tendons, the intermediate dorsal cutaneus branch of the superficial peroneal nerve, the tibiotalar joint line and the often visible greater saphenous vein.

- The intermediate dorsal cutaneous branch of the superficial peroneal nerve can usually be identified prior to placement of the anterolateral portal, reducing risk of nerve injury.

- The superficial peroneal nerve divides into the intermediate and medial dorsal cutaneous branches approximately 6.5 cm proximal to the tip of the fibula with the intermediate branch overlying the superficial extensor retinaculum, traversing the extensor tendons between the third and fourth metatarsals. The medial dorsal cutaneous branch crosses the anterior aspect of the ankle joint superficial to the extensor tendons, lateral and parallel to the extensor hallucis longus (EHL) tendon.

- The dorsalis pedis artery is palpable throughout its course anteriorly and at the level of the ankle joint; it resides between the tibialis anterior tendon and the extensor hallucis longus tendon. It courses deep to the EHL tendon as it migrates toward the great toe medially.

- The peroneus tertius tendon is palpable at the level of the ankle joint as the lateral border of the common extensors, lateral to the EHL tendon

- When entering the joint, recall that the dome of the talus is convex and the plafond of the tibia is slightly concave.

Portals

- Careful placement of vertical incisions **through skin only** can be performed with a 15-blade scalpel to minimize the risk of injury to superficial nerves.
- Deeper layers should be penetrated bluntly with the use of a straight mosquito clamp to enter the joint, followed by a blunt obturator.
- The safest portals are the anterolateral, anteromedial and posterolateral portals and these are the most commonly used.
- The anteromedial portal
  - Often created first because it is typically the easiest and safest (risks are the greater saphenous vein and nerve, which are on average 9 mm and 7.4 mm medial to the portal site)
  - It is recommended to distend the joint initially with 10 to 15 mL of saline or lactated Ringer (LR) solution before making portals to minimize the risk of damaging intra-articular structures and to move the periarticular nerves away from the joint.

- Insert an 18- to 20-gauge needle just medial to the tibialis anterior tendon at the level of the joint line or slightly proximal and inject 10 to 15 mL sterile saline or LR solution to distend the ankle joint.

- After the joint is distended, the needle is removed and a superficial vertical incision is made, centered on the needle entry site.

- Through this portal the arthroscope cannula with blunt trocar can be introduced and then the arthroscope exchanged for the trocar and the joint can be infused with saline through the side port on the cannula.

- **The anterolateral portal**
  - At risk are the branches of the superficial peroneal nerve with an average distance of 6.2 mm from the nearest branch to the portal site
    - Identify this nerve by plantarflexing fourth toe to put the nerve on stretch. The nerve may also be visualized with transillumination of the skin and subcutaneous tissue with the scope camera light (see later).
  - Can be made under arthroscopic visualization for improved accuracy and be modified slightly depending on identified pathology
  - This portal is made just lateral to the peroneus tertius tendon at the tibiotalar joint line.
  - A 1.5-inch 25-gauge needle is used to identify the portal site, and confirmation of its location at an optimal entry location can be visualized with the arthroscope.
  - The skin can be transilluminated with the arthroscope to help avoid the neurovascular structures by bringing the arthroscope to the capsule at the anterolateral joint, reducing the room lights, and looking for the tendons and nerves through the illuminated skin.

- **The posterolateral portal**
  - This portal site is on average 6 mm posterior to the sural nerve and 9.5 mm posterior to the lesser saphenous vein.
  - Needle localization and arthroscopic visualization is recommended to assist in placement, using the arthroscope in either the anterolateral or anteromedial portal.
  - This portal is made just lateral to the Achilles tendon approximately 1.5 cm proximal to the distal tip of the fibula, placing the needle at a 45-degree angle aiming toward the medial malleolus.

- Other described portals and at-risk structures
  - Anterocentral
    - Between the tendons of the extensor digitorum communis
    - Dorsalis pedis artery and deep peroneal nerve at risk
    - Use of this portal discouraged due to neurovascular risk
  - Posteromedial
    - Used during posterior ankle arthroscopy. See later for details
- Posterocentral (trans-Achilles)
  - Through Achilles tendon and inferior to joint line
  - Not recommended due to morbidity to the Achilles tendon

Diagnostic Arthroscopy Technique

- A thorough diagnostic evaluation should be undertaken in a systematic format to allow for reproducible documentation and accuracy of diagnosis.
- The specific order of evaluation is surgeon-dependent but should be completed in a systematic fashion.
- A 21-step examination has been described by Ferkel and colleagues as a guideline to evaluate all aspects of the ankle joint.
  - Anterior
    - Deltoid ligament
    - Medial gutter
    - Medial talus
    - Central talus
    - Lateral talus
    - Trifurcation of talus, tibia, and fibula
    - Lateral gutter
    - Anterior gutter
  - Central
    - Medial tibia and talus
    - Central tibia and talus
    - Lateral tibiofibular or talofibular articulation
    - Posterior inferior tibiofibular ligament

▸ Transverse ligament

▸ Reflection of flexor hallucis longus

■ Posterior

▸ Posteromedial gutter

▸ Posteromedial talus

▸ Posterocentral talus

▸ Posterolateral talus

▸ Posterior talofibular articulation

▸ Posterolateral gutter

▸ Posterior gutter

- Begin with gentle distraction of the ankle joint.
- Enter the joint through the intended location for the anteromedial portal with an 18- to 20-gauge needle and inject 10 to 15 mL of saline or LR solution.
- Make a small vertical incision through skin only, centering over injection site.
- Use a straight mosquito clamp to bluntly penetrate the capsule and enter the joint. This can also be used to gently widen the portal.
- Then place the arthroscopic cannula with blunt obturator.
- Remove the obturator and place the 30-degree arthroscope into the cannula and begin the diagnostic arthroscopy.
- The anterolateral portal can be made by aiming the arthroscope toward the intended entry site and transilluminating the skin to help avoid nerves and veins with the localizing needle and the incision.
- An 18- to 20-gauge needle can be used to penetrate in the intended location and, with the use of the arthroscope, the ideal location can be verified before making the incision *(Fig. 4-3)*.
- Again the incision is vertical and through skin only, following the same steps as the initial portal, visualizing entry with the arthroscope.
- Depending on the identified pathology and procedures to be performed, the posterolateral portal may be created in the same format.

Positioning Pearls

- Joint distraction, while providing more space between the tibia and talus, will often reduce the overall working area as it places tension on the capsule.
- Dorsiflexion will allow more working area in the anterior aspect of the ankle joint as the capsule is relaxed. This also places the major portion of the weight-bearing articular surface under the protection of the tibial plafond, and can allow safer entry into the capsule for placing instruments.

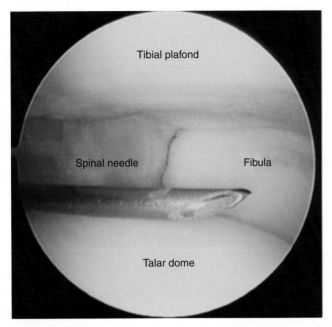

Figure 4-3. Arthroscopic image of the ankle joint from the anteromedial portal, using needle localization to safely create the anterolateral working portal.

- Plantar flexion will increase the posterior working area as the capsule relaxes, at the expense of decreasing the anterior working space with capsular tension.
- These principles can be used to maximize the safe working area for the given location of pathology being treated.
- In general, the anterior working space is disproportionately larger than the posterior space and is largely due to a large anterior capsular recess, but this is variable between patients and with foot position.

Common Procedures

Anterior Ankle Bony Impingement ("Footballer's Ankle") (Fig. 4-4A-E)

- Bony impingement anteriorly with decreased dorsiflexion typically with osteophyte formation on anterior tibial plafond that abuts the neck of talus, which may result in notch formation or bony spur formation on the talus
- Most common in dancers, and soccer, basketball, or football players
- Results from anterior capsular strain due to forced plantar flexion with calcific deposits or repetitive dorsiflexion leading to subchondral injury to talar neck with osteophyte formation
- May also develop in the chronically unstable ankle.

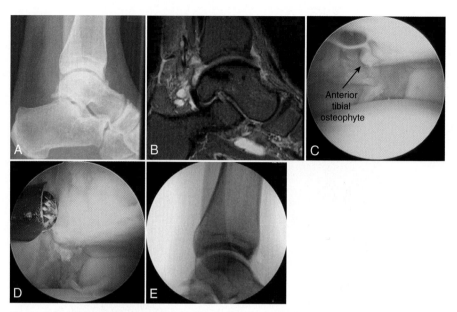

Figure 4-4. A. Preoperative lateral radiograph of a patient treated by the senior author with anterior tibiotalar impingement. **B.** Preoperative sagittal MRI with further detail of the impingement anteriorly at the ankle joint line. **C.** Arthroscopic image from the anteromedial portal demonstrating the anterior osteophyte on the distal tibia (*arrow*). **D.** Arthroscopic image of the resection of the osteophyte using a partially hooded high-speed burr. **E.** Intraoperative fluoroscopy image documenting the resection of the anterior osteophytes.

- May occur in conjunction with synovitis or anterolateral impingement processes

- Treatment is focused on gentle elevation of the anterior capsule from the tibia and talus with resection of the bony prominence.

- Technique

  - Standard anterolateral and anteromedial portals are used as described.

  - The 30-degree arthroscope and a 3.5-mm aggressive shaver or 4.0-mm high-speed burr can be used for resection of the bony prominence.

  - Requires careful use of suction to avoid collapse of the capsular window of working space, and often visualization and working space is improved without the use of traction

  - The capsule can be gently reflected with the shaver used as a probe or an accessory portal can be made and a switching stick, Freer elevator, or probe is used as a retractor on the anterior capsule.

  - The anterior neurovascular structures are at risk as they are adjacent to the anterior capsule, and at risk with aggressive shaving of the anterior soft tissue; therefore keep the shaver or burr facing bone at all times.

■ Further, anterior synovectomy using a radiofrequency device is generally discouraged due to the risk of thermal injury to the anterior neurovascular structures.

■ Identify the normal margin of the talus and tibia (both medial and lateral) to identify the resection level and débride the prominence back to this level, working completely across the joint for a full and equal resection.

■ The resection can be verified with dorsiflexion of the ankle with the arthroscope in the anterior capsular recess to visualize the motion.

■ Fluoroscopy may be used to confirm the level and adequacy of resection.

Ankle Synovitis/Anterolateral Impingement *(Fig. 4-5A,B)*

● Synovitis is often present with the complaint of global ankle pain and is certainly associated with multiple pathologies.

● Arthroscopic treatment of synovitis alone is indicated only if all conservative measures fail, or if it is present in addition to other pathology that warrants arthroscopy.

● Anterolateral impingement is typically due to soft tissue scar impingement that develops after fracture or significant ankle sprains and develops in the anterolateral gutter, below the syndesmosis.

● Maximal dorsiflexion with deep palpation to the anterolateral aspect of the ankle joint will reproduce the pain.

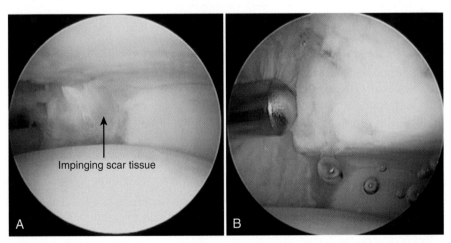

Figure 4-5. A. Arthroscopic image from the anteromedial portal demonstrating the thickened scar tissue present in anterolateral impingement. **B.** Débridement of the scar tissue in anterolateral impingement with an oscillating shaver.

- Treatment of these lesions is similar to that described for anterior impingement, except that the soft tissue may be débrided with the shaver or radiofrequency/electrothermal device.
- Technique
  - The hypertrophic and inflamed synovium may be debrided using the 3.5-mm shaver, but careful use of suction is critical to avoid over-resection or collapse of the working space.
  - Inflamed and hemorrhagic synovium may require radiofrequency ablation or coagulation as well.
  - Care should be taken to use low power settings with the radiofrequency or electrothermal device, especially when working off the anterior capsule.
  - Débridement of synovium should include the anterior joint line and both medial and lateral gutters, which may require alternately working and viewing portals for completeness.
  - The capsule itself should not be violated in the débridement.
  - The soft tissue impingement lesion is typically a thick whitish scar tissue, which may be meniscoid in quality and appearance and may represent hypertrophy of the anterior tibiofibular ligament.
  - This may require the use of ablators and biters in addition to shavers for resection.
  - After resection, a final inspection should be made and hemostasis obtained which can be augmented by evaluating without inflow and the tourniquet (if used) deflated.

Osteochondral Lesions of the Talus *(Fig. 4-6A-E)*

- Typically the result of trauma
  - Lateral talar dome more commonly involved in acute trauma with dorsiflexion and inversion and occurs in the anterolateral corner of the dome.
  - Medial lesions tend to be more posterior and result from chronic impaction of the posteromedial talar dome against the tibial plafond with combined inversion, plantar flexion, and external rotation forces.
  - Medial lesions tend to be deeper lesions, whereas the lateral lesions are often thin.
- Depending on the lesion characteristics, these can be treated with microfracture, repair, or retrograde drilling.

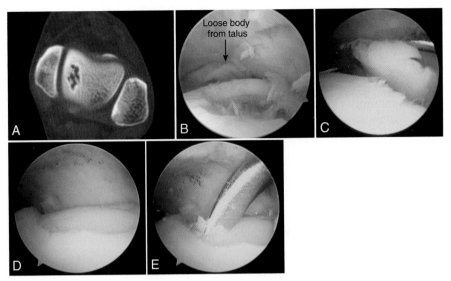

Figure 4-6. A. Axial CT scan image demonstrating an OCD (osteochondritis dissecans) lesion of the dome of the talus. **B.** Arthroscopic image demonstrating the OCD lesion in the talar dome with a loose body in the gutter. **C.** A superficial (cartilage only) and unstable chondral lesion of the talar dome. **D.** Arthroscopic image after débridement of the chondral injury leaving an exposed focal area of subchondral bone on the talar dome. **E.** Introduction of a microfracture awl into the periphery of the débrided lesion.

- **If microfracture is chosen, the nonviable cartilage is removed with the combination of shavers, curettes, and graspers to expose the underlying bone.**

  - If an isolated chondral lesion is identified, all calcified cartilage must also be removed.

  - If an osteochondral lesion is present, fibrous tissue must be removed from the bony bed before microfracture or drilling.

    - A firm rim of healthy viable cartilage must be present and the underlying bone must be débrided to a healthy bleeding bed of bone.

    - Microfracture awls are then introduced perpendicular to the bone surface around the perimeter of the lesion and centrally, spacing apart by 3 to 4 mm.

    - Occasionally, the osteochondral lesion cannot be drilled or microfractured through the standard portals. In this situation, some surgeons will drill through the malleolus into the lesion. An ACL drill guide can be used to serve as a guide to improve accuracy with the transmalleolar drilling of the talus.

    - The bed is then débrided with the shaver and punctate bleeding and marrow contents should be visualized after stopping the inflow.

▶ If a viable osteochondral flap is identified and repair is chosen, standard arthroscopic technique using anteromedial and anterolateral portals can be used, with accessory portals used as needed for fixation.

- The flap can be elevated with the blunt-tipped probe and the underlying bony bed can be débrided as necessary with a curette or shaver to allow for a healthy bed for the flap to heal into.

- Repair can be completed in retrograde fashion with Kirschner wire fixation percutaneously, with wires cut externally for later removal.

- Antegrade repair can also be performed with bioabsorbable pins or screws sunken below the chondral surface.

▶ In situ, nondisplaced fragments can be treated with retrograde drilling using standard arthroscopy to verify the location and integrity of the lesion.

- With an intact cartilage cap, the drilling procedure may be considered.

- Cannulated systems for retrograde drilling are available and can be placed through a small incision at the sinus tarsi combined with fluoroscopy to confirm the correct placement.

- A guidewire can be placed under fluoroscopic guidance to the level of subchondral bone, over which the cannulated drill is advanced.

- The arthroscope can be used to visualize the cartilage cap to verify that its integrity is maintained.

Arthroscopic Ankle Arthrodesis

- Offers many advantages over open technique: less invasive, more rapid recovery, less soft tissue dissection

- Indicated for pain caused by post-traumatic, degenerative, or inflammatory arthritis that is not responsive to conservative therapy.

- Beneficial for patients with wound healing problems, such as patients with peripheral vascular disease, dermatological problems, or rheumatoid arthritis.

- Contraindications to the procedure include varus or valgus deformities of more than 15 degrees, anteroposterior deformity of more than 15 degrees, significant joint incongruity, or bony destruction due to osteonecrosis.

- Resection of the articular cartilage and subchondral bone from the tibial plafond, the dome of the talus, and the medial and lateral gutters is essential.

- The ankle should be aligned in neutral position with approximately 5 degrees of heel valgus. Adequate bone purchase by screw fixation is necessary for compression and stabilization during the fusion process.
- Variable union rates have been reported in the literature.
- Posterolateral portal required to sufficiently prepare posterior aspect of joint.
- Technique
  - Use positioning, set-up, and instruments described earlier.
  - Anteromedial, anterolateral, and posterolateral portals are used. The posterolateral portal is used for inflow and for viewing during posterior débridement.
  - Use a shaver to remove the soft tissue to expose the joint, both malleoli, and both medial and lateral gutters.
  - With a full-radius resector and abrader, remove the articular cartilage, beginning from the medial malleolus and talus, moving around the lateral side of the ankle, and ending as far posteriorly as can be seen. Use caution not to distort the normal architecture of the talus or tibial plafond.
  - While visualizing through the posterolateral portal, use a small, curved resector or rasp to remove the posterior tissues through the anterior portals. If necessary, the arthroscope can be placed anteriorly and the instruments can be placed posteriorly.
  - Once débridement is complete, a small burr is used to prepare the joint surface, expose subchondral bone, and maximize bleeding surface area. Bone graft can be inserted if indicated.
  - Traction is removed, the joint is reduced, and alignment is confirmed on fluoroscopy. Use the standard percutaneous three-screw configuration for fixation (with 6.5- to 7.3-mm cannulated screws), holding the joint in a compressed, reduced position while tightening the screws. Direct the screws into the middle of the body of the talus without violating the subtalar joint.
  - Verify correct alignment and reduction of the joint on lateral radiographs.

Posterior Ankle Arthroscopy
- Performed in the prone position
- Distraction often not necessary to achieve diagnostic and therapeutic goals
- Indications
  - Débridement of posterior tibio-talar joint
  - Removal of loose bodies

- Treatment of articular pathology (OCD) in posterior third of joint

- Removal of symptomatic os trigonum

- Tenolysis or débridement of FHL tendon

- Resection of Haglund deformity with limited débridement of insertional Achilles tendinosis

• Posterolateral portal created first, as described earlier.

• Needle localization and fluoroscopy may be used to confirm level.

• Posteromedial portal

  - Placed immediately medial to the Achilles tendon just inferior to the joint line. Level can be confirmed by visualization with fluoroscopy or with scope camera placed via posterolateral portal.

  - Use extreme caution because tibial nerve is about 6 to 10 mm medial to the portal site.

  - Direct needle and all instruments with a lateral angle (i.e., toward the lateral gutter) to avoid the neurovascular bundle.

  - Always be aware of the location of the FHL as an indicator of the neurovascular bundle.

Subtalar Joint Arthroscopy *(Fig. 4-7)*

• Prone or lateral position

• Invasive or noninvasive distraction methods can be helpful.

• Indications

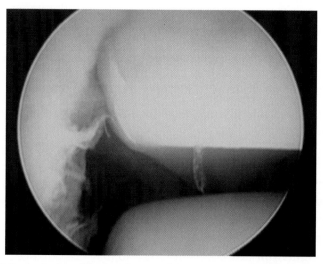

Figure 4-7. Arthroscopic view of the lateral gutter of the subtalar joint with the talus above and the calcaneous below.

- Posterior arthroscopic subtalar arthrodesis (PASTA) (see Lee et al. in references)

- Evaluation of posterior facet reduction during fixation of calcaneus fracture

- Débridement/synovectomy of posterior facet and anterior portion of the posterior subtalar joint

- Débridement of sinus tarsi (for sinus tarsi syndrome)

- Release of adhesions

- Portal placement

  - As in posterior ankle arthroscopy, anteromedial and anterolateral portals placed immediately adjacent to the Achilles tendon and directed away from the neurovascular structures

  - Starting point just superior to subtalar joint line

  - Instruments directed at slightly downward angle in line with the subtalar joint

  - An accessory lateral portal (1 cm proximal and 1 cm posterior to the tip of the lateral malleolus) has been described for distraction by inserting a large blunt trocar into the subtalar joint (see Lee et al.)

  - Fluoroscopic guidance may be useful.

Tendoscopy

- Smaller arthroscopic instruments allow evaluation and limited treatment of tendons in the foot and ankle.
- At present, there are limited data on these techniques.
- Described endoscopic techniques include

  - Peroneal tendon disorders

  - FHL impingement, adhesions, or tendon degeneration

  - Repair of Achilles ruptures

  - Débridement of Achilles tendinopathy

  - Inflammatory and degenerative processes of the posterior tibial tendon

- Portals for tendoscopy of the peroneals (prone position)

  - Distal portal is made first at approximately 2.0 cm distal to the posterior border of the lateral malleolus

  - The tendon sheath can be identified after a small incision is made in the skin.

  - The sheath is then penetrated with a 2.7-mm, 30-degree arthroscope

- A proximal portal can then be created at approximately 2.0 cm proximal to the tip of the lateral malleolus at the posterior border after localizing with a spinal needle under arthroscopic visualization.

- Evaluation of the tendons should include as far proximal as approximately 6 cm from the tip of the lateral malleolus where the two tendons are separated by a thin membrane into two compartments.

- Through these portals, a full diagnostic evaluation is possible, in addition to groove-deepening procedures for peroneal stability, débridement of tears, and performing a partial or total synovectomy.

- Portals for tendoscopy of the Achilles tendon (prone position)
  - Distal portal is again typically made first and is along the lateral border of the Achilles tendon at approximately 2 cm distal to the site of pathology.

  - A skin incision is made followed by a mosquito clamp to carefully widen the soft tissue, followed by placement of the 2.7-mm, 30-degree arthroscope.

  - A proximal portal is then created with spinal needle localization as previously described.

  - This proximal portal may be created along the medial border of the tendon, typically 2 to 4 cm above the level of the pathology for a more complete evaluation.

- Portals for tendoscopy of the posterior tibialis tendon (supine position)
  - The posterior edge of the medial malleolus is the key landmark for the two primary portals.

  - The distal portal is typically made first at approximately 2.0 cm distal to the posterior aspect of the tip of the medial malleolus with the same technique as previously described.

  - The proximal portal is made at approximately 2 to 4 cm proximal to the posterior edge of the tip of the medial malleolus using spinal needle guidance into the tendon sheath.

Complications

- Variable reports on ankle arthroscopy complications from <1% to 17%
- Majority of complications are neurologic injury either from incisions for portals (especially anterolateral portal) or from distraction.

- ■ Risk factors identified for neurologic injury include prolonged distraction times, deep incisions when making portals, and repeated passes or multiple attempts at passage of instruments through portals

- Other risk factors for complications include portals placed too close together leading to skin necrosis, tendon injury from portal placement, damage to the capsule and ligaments from excessive débridement, excessive extravasation of fluid into the soft tissue from capsular disruption, or damage with repeated attempts at inflow trocar placement.

- Sinus tract formation has been reported from delayed healing of traumatized portal sites or postoperative infection. Persistent draining fluid should be cultured, wounds evaluated for need of débridement, and the joint temporarily immobilized to allow healing.

- Iatrogenic damage to chondral surfaces may be under-reported.

- Deep vein thrombi can occur, but are rare. At-risk patients should receive consideration for DVT prophylaxis when appropriate.

- Adherence to meticulous surgical technique and standard arthroscopic protocols is imperative.

REFERENCES

Bulstra GH, Olsthoorn PGM, and van Dijk CN. Tendoscopy of the posterior tibial tendon. *Foot Ankle Clin N Am* 2006; 11:421–427.

Cheng JC and Ferkel RD. The role of arthroscopy in ankle and subtalar degenerative joint disease. *Clin Ortho Rel Res* 1998; 349:65–72.

Ferkel RD, Heath DD, and Guhl JF. Neurologic complications of ankle arthroscopy. *Arthroscopy* 1996; 12(2):200–208.

Ferkel RD, Small HN, and Gittins JE. Complications in foot and ankle arthroscopy. *Clin Ortho Rel Res* 2001; 391:89–104.

Hyer CF, Buchanan MM, Philbin TM, et al. Ankle arthroscopy. In ElAttrache NS, Harner CD, Mirzayan R, and Sekiya JK (eds). *Surgical Techniques in Sports Medicine*, Philadelphia, Lippincott, Williams and Wilkins, 2007; pp 657–671.

Golano P, Vega J, Perez-Carro L, and Gotzens V. Ankle anatomy for the arthroscopist. Part I: The portals. *Foot Ankle Clin N Am* 2006; 11:253–273.

Golano P, Vega J, Perez-Carro L, and Gotzens V. Ankle anatomy for the arthroscopist. Part II: Role of the ankle ligaments in soft tissue impingement. *Foot Ankle Clin N Am* 2006; 11:275–296.

Lee KB, Saltzman CL, Suh JS, et al. A posterior 3-portal arthroscopic approach for isolated subtalar arthrodesis. *Arthroscopy* 2008; 24(11):1306–1310.

Lui TH. Ankle arthroscopy with patient in prone position. *Arch Orthop Trauma Surg* 2008; 128:1283–1285.

Scholten PE and van Dijk CN. Tendoscopy of the peroneal tendons. *Foot Ankle Clin N Am* 2006; 11:415–420.

Steenstra F and van Dijk CN. Achilles tendoscopy. *Foot Ankle Clin N Am* 2006; 11:429–438.

Stetson WB and Ferkel RD. Ankle arthroscopy: I. Technique and complications. *J Amer Acad Ortho Surg* 1996; 4:17–23.

Stetson WB and Ferkel RD. Ankle arthroscopy: II. Indications and results. *J Amer Acad Ortho Surg* 1996; 4:24–34.

Van Dijk CN and Van Bergen CJA. Advancements in ankle arthroscopy. *J Amer Acad Ortho Surg* 2008; 16:635–646.

CHAPTER 5

SHOULDER ARTHROSCOPY

Melissa D. Willenborg, Mark D. Miller and
Marc R. Safran

Introduction

- The modern era of management of shoulder pathology began in the 1930s
  with the work of Codman.
  - Significant contributions to understanding of rotator cuff
    pathology originated with Neer, whereas Bankart and Rowe
    were the major proponents of concepts underlying the current
    understanding of shoulder instability.
  - The management of shoulder arthritis in the modern era is
    credited to Neer.
- Arthroscopy of the shoulder did not become routine practice until the 1980s.
- Since that time, developments in technology have led to routine use of
  arthroscopy for diagnosis and treatment of several different pathologic
  conditions of the shoulder.
- Ongoing technologic advances ensure that shoulder arthroscopy will
  continue to evolve as a treatment modality for shoulder disorders.

Preoperative Considerations

- Review all pertinent medical records and perform a thorough history and
  physical examination prior to the procedure and obtain appropriate imaging
  to confirm the diagnosis and to reduce the risk of surprises.
  - Preoperative consultation with appropriate primary care or
    medical specialists and anesthesiologists to decrease
    perioperative risk of complications
- Anesthesia can consist of general, general with regional nerve blocks, or
  regional anesthesia alone.
  - General anesthesia is usually chosen in combination with a
    regional nerve block for patient comfort during and after the
    procedure.

- Regional nerve blocks give longer pain relief postoperatively. Regional anesthesia alone, however, usually is poorly tolerated when the procedure is performed in the lateral decubitus position.

- Hypotensive anesthesia aids in visualization during the procedure and reduces blood loss.

- **Examination under anesthesia (EUA)**
  - Should be performed on every patient prior to beginning the procedure

  - Systematic examination should be performed including evaluation of range of motion (ROM) and stability of the shoulder.

- **Positioning**
  - Lateral decubitus *(Fig. 5-1)*

    ▸ In the supine position, the patient undergoes general anesthesia and an examination under anesthesia is performed.

    ▸ The patient is placed in the lateral decubitus position using a bean bag, often rotated backward 20 degrees. An axillary roll is used to protect the brachial plexus and padding is placed between the down leg and table, as well as between the knees, as all bony prominences must be well padded.

    ▸ Most arthroscopists will place the arm in a sterile traction device with the arm in 45 to 70 degrees of abduction and 20 to 30 degrees of forward flexion. A 10 to 15 lbs of traction is usually adequate.

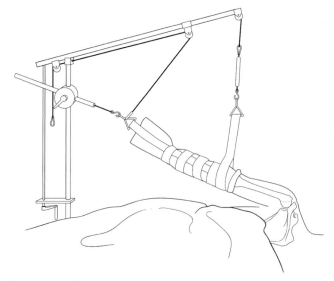

Figure 5-1. The lateral decubitus position for shoulder arthroscopy. *(Courtesy of Arthrex, Naples, Florida.)*

▸ All arthroscopic shoulder procedures can be performed from this position, with posterior shoulder stabilization a little easier in the lateral decubitus position.

▸ Higher risk of neuropraxia has been documented as a result of traction.

▸ Conversion to an open procedure may require repositioning and redraping the patient.

▸ Regional anesthesia by itself is often not well tolerated in this position.

■ Beach chair *(Fig. 5-2)*

▸ Patient is placed supine and an examination under anesthesia is performed in this position.

▸ The patient is then placed in a beach chair position as seen in Figure 5-2.

▸ Be careful to monitor the blood pressure while the patient is being brought up into the beach chair position.

▸ Be careful of the neck position and head support when positioning the patient

▸ Protect the elbow/ulnar nerve of both arms as they may have pressure depending on how they are held during the arthroscopy.

▸ Easier for anesthesia control during surgery

▸ Position makes conversion to open procedure easier.

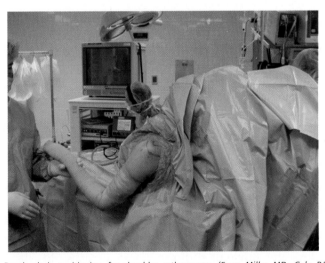

Figure 5-2. Beach chair positioning for shoulder arthroscopy. *(From Miller MD, Cole BJ. Textbook of Arthroscopy. Philadelphia, Elsevier, 2004 [Fig. 8-2B, p 67].)*

- General anesthesia with regional nerve blocks or regional alone can be tolerated.

- Risk of cerebral hypoperfusion with hypotensive anesthesia as well as the small risk of air embolism

- Difficulty performing posterior stabilization

- Easier to perform dynamic assessment (no traction to remove from the arm)

- **Equipment**
  - Arthroscope
    - 30-degree arthroscope most commonly used
    - 70-degree arthroscope useful for access to anterior labrum/glenoid, inferior glenohumeral ligament and sub-coracoid region.
  - Cannulas
    - Decrease fluid extravasation into the surrounding soft tissue
    - Maintain portal position without the need to create new portal sites and thus create undue soft tissue trauma
    - Necessary for arthroscopic knot-tying to reduce the risk of capturing unwanted soft tissue in the knot
  - Instruments
    - Full complement of shoulder instruments has been devised to aid in the performing of procedures for manipulation and/or repair of soft tissues
      - Arthroscopic soft tissue graspers
      - Arthroscopic curettes
      - Arthroscopic biters
      - Arthroscopic rasps
      - Arthroscopic microfracture awls
      - Arthroscopic soft tissue–penetrating, suture-passing or grasping devices
      - Arthroscopic suture-passing devices
      - Arthroscopic suture-management cannulas
      - Arthroscopic shavers
      - Arthroscopic burrs
      - Underwater Bovie or radiofrequency devices aid with visualization during the procedure by allowing coagulation or soft tissue ablation.

- Arthroscopic suture anchors
- Arthroscopic tacks

Relevant Anatomy *(Fig. 5-3)*

- Glenohumeral joint
  - Greatest range of motion of any joint at the expense of stability
  - Static restraints are the bony anatomy, glenoid labrum, ligaments, and capsule. The dynamic restraints are the muscles about the shoulder, the negative-pressure system, and adhesion-cohesion.

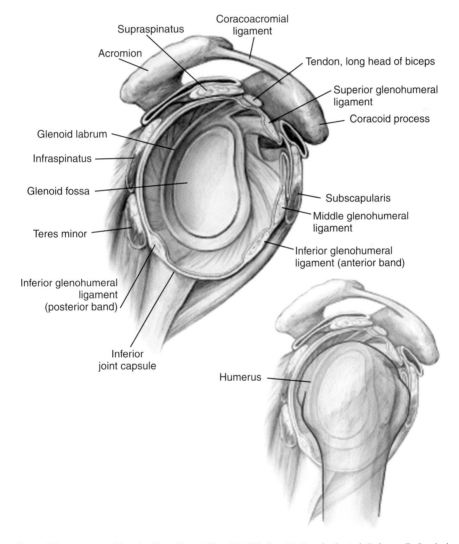

Figure 5-3. Anatomy of the shoulder. *(From Miller MD, Chhabra AB, Hurwitz S, et al. Orthopaedic Surgical Approaches. Philadelphia, Elsevier, 2008 [Fig. SA-4, p 13].)*

▶ Rotator interval (RI)

- Area of the capsule between the subscapularis inferiorly and the supraspinatus superiorly

- The coracoid forms the medial base and the transverse humeral ligament forms the lateral apex.

- The contents of the RI are the biceps tendon, coracohumeral ligament (CHL) and superior glenohumeral ligament (SGHL)

▶ Labrum

- Deepens the joint

- Increases the surface area

- Anchors glenohumeral ligament complex

- Varying anatomy and shapes

- Anterosuperior labrum may not be attached, and this normal variant is known as a sublabral foramen.

▶ Glenoid

- Pear shaped with average of 5 degrees of upward tilt and between 7 degrees of retroversion to 10 degrees of anteversion

- There is a bare area in the middle of the glenoid, halfway between the anterior and posterior borders of the glenoid.

▶ Ligaments

- Thickenings in the capsule.

- **Superior glenohumeral ligament (SGHL)**

  - The SGHL and coraco-humeral ligament (CHL) resist inferior translation and external rotation with the arm in adduction. They also resist posterior translation with the arm flexed forward, adducted, and internally rotated.

  - Superior glenohumeral ligament has two sites of origin: the coracoid and the supraglenoid tubercle—just anterior to the long head of biceps origin on the superior labrum. Its insertion is on the proximal lesser tuberosity.

  - Origin of the CHL is extra-articular on the lateral surface of coracoid. The CHL insertion is the greater and lesser tuberosities spanning the bicipital groove.

- **Middle glenohumeral ligament (MGHL)**

  - Most variable anatomy

  - Absent in as many as 30% of patients

- Resists external rotation when the arm is abducted and anterior/posterior translation of the arm at 45 degrees of abduction and external rotation

- Origin is the anatomic of the proximal humerus neck and insertion is the labrum.

- Inferior glenohumeral ligament (IGHL)

  - The PRIMARY RESTRAINT to anterior, posterior, and interior translation of the joint with the arm elevated 45 to 90 degrees

  - Origin is anterior inferior labrum

  - Anterior band limits anterior translation in external rotation and abduction.

  - The posterior band limits posterior humeral head translation in abduction and internal rotation

  - The area between the anterior and posterior bands, known as the axillary pouch, may function as a hammock, holding the humeral head.

  - Dynamic restraints are the biceps tendon, rotator cuff, and surrounding musculature.

    ‣ Rotator cuff muscle acts to depress and compress the convex humeral head against the concave glenoid.

      • Subscapularis inserts on the lesser tuberosity.

      • Supraspinatus, infraspinatus, and teres minor insert on the greater tuberosity.

    ‣ Internal rotators of the shoulder are the pectoralis major, latissimus dorsi, and subscapularis.

    ‣ External rotators are the teres minor and infraspinatus.

    ‣ The biceps tendon is located in the Rotator Interval as described earlier and its function in stabilization is still debated.

      • The biceps is the lighthouse of the arthroscopic anatomy of the shoulder.

      • The biceps inserts into the superior labrum.

    ‣ The supraspinatus tendon inserts on the articular margin of the greater tuberosity over a distance of 12 to 18 mm.

    ‣ The bare area is the area of the posterosuperior humeral head just posterior to the supraspinatus insertion where the rotator cuff does not attach to the articular margin and there is exposed bone and no articular cartilage.

- Acromioclavicular joint

  - Gliding joint with fibrocartilaginous disc.

  - Acromioclavicular (AC) ligament prevents anteroposterior translation of the distal clavicle.

  - Coracoclavicular (conoid and trapezoid) ligament prevents superior displacement of the distal clavicle (actually the clavicle and coracoclavicular ligaments prevent drooping of the scapula [acromion]).

  - The AC joint does contribute to shoulder motion.

Portal Placement *(Fig. 5-4)*

- Posterior portal

  - 1 to 2 cm distal and 1 to 2 cm medial to the posterolateral corner of the acromion

  - This varies somewhat with position of the patient and type of procedure.

  - Verify position with spinal needle prior to incision.

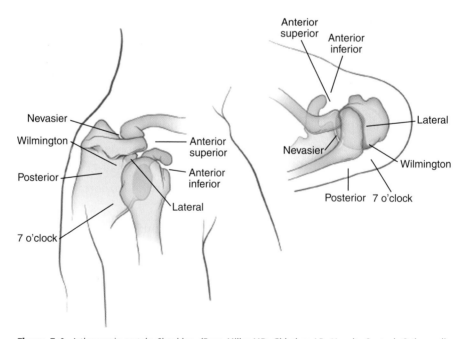

Figure 5-4. Arthroscopic portals: Shoulder. *(From Miller MD, Chhabra AB, Hurwitz S, et al. Orthopaedic Surgical Approaches. Philadelphia, Elsevier, 2008 [Fig. SA-48, p 54].)*

- Primary viewing portal
- Pierces posterior deltoid muscle and travels in the interval between the infraspinatus and the teres minor
- The axillary nerve and suprascapular nerve are at risk with this portal, but are relatively safe.

- Anterior superior portal
  - Superior and lateral to the coracoid—just anterior to the AC joint
  - Localized with spinal needle in an outside-in technique just anterior to the biceps tendon next to the superior glenoid
  - Can be moved more medially for a distal clavicle excision
  - Primarily an instrument portal but can be used to visualize the anterior glenoid rim and labrum, the posterior joint, as well as to visualize internal impingement dynamically
  - Pierces the anterior deltoid and travels through the rotator interval, avoiding injury to the rotator cuff
  - Neurovascular structures at risk include the musculocutaneous nerve, axillary nerve, as well as the cephalic vein, brachial plexus, and axillary artery

- Anterior inferior portal
  - Lateral to the coracoid
  - Pierces anterior deltoid muscle and enters joint just above subscapularis
  - If too low, risk of injury to the axillary nerve
  - If too medial, risk of injury to musculocutaneous nerve (1.5 to 4 cm)
  - Minimal risk of injury to cephalic vein, brachial plexus, and axillary artery

- Lateral portal
  - 1 to 2 cm distal to the acromion
  - Either mid acromion (anterior to posterior) or junction of the (anterior third, posterior two-thirds)
  - Localized with spinal needle while viewing subacromial space
  - Used for subacromial decompression and rotator cuff repairs
  - Can be extended for mini-open deltoid splitting rotator cuff repairs
  - Pierces middle deltoid muscle

- Axillary nerve at risk, because this averages 5 to 6 cm from the lateral acromial border, but may be as close as 3 cm from the acromion
- Posteroinferior portal
  - 2 cm above the posterior axillary fold
  - Used as inflow portal
  - Dangerous portal due to proximity of the axillary nerve, posterior humeral circumflex artery, and suprascapular nerve
- Posterolateral portal (Wilmington)
  - 1 cm anterior and 1 cm distal to the posterolateral corner of the acromion
  - Localized with spinal needle while viewing the superior labrum
  - Used for instrumentation during a superior labral anterior to posterior (SLAP) repair
- Anteroinferior portal
  - Inferior and lateral to the coracoid
  - Localized with spinal needle using outside-in technique superior to the subscapularis
  - Used primarily for instrumentation for anterior Bankhart repair suture anchor placement
- Supraspinatus (Nevasier) portal
  - Corner of the supraspinatus fossa
  - Localize with spinal needle
  - Enters joint just medial to the supraglenoid tubercle
  - Used for SLAP and rotator cuff repairs
  - Suprascapular nerve and artery are 3 cm medial to portal.

Diagnostic Arthroscopy

- Scope insertion
  - The posterior portal site is made with a No. 11 blade scalpel after the joint is localized with a spinal needle. The joint can be insufflated with 40 to 60 mL of normal saline prior to incision. The scalpel, just like the spinal needle, is directed anteromedially toward the coracoid.
  - A blunt trocar and sheath is then introduced along the path of the incision, toward the coracoid, which is located anteriorly and medially toward the joint line.

- The glenoid rim may be palpated and entry into the joint is just lateral to this point.

- Intra-articular position is confirmed with return of joint fluid through the trocar.

- The camera is then introduced to inspect the joint. Inspection starts at the base of the biceps and continues clockwise to inspect the glenoid, labrum, and rotator cuff.

- The anterior superior portal is then made for instrumentation and palpation of the structures. This is done using a spinal needle and outside-in technique.

- Glenohumeral articulation
  - The joint surface is examined by internally and externally rotating the arm.

  - A small cartilage deficit on the central portion of the glenoid (bare area) is a normal finding.

  - In a beach chair position, the camera is directed upward.

- Biceps tendon/superior labrum
  - A probe is inserted into the anterior portal and the biceps tendon and superior labral complex are probed for stability.

  - A Bovie can be introduced through the anterior portal to perform a biceps tenotomy if necessary.

  - The scope is then advanced anteriorly to inspect the path of the biceps tendon for synovitis or fraying. The probe is used to pull the biceps tendon that normally sits in the bicipital groove into view.

- Anterior capsule/SGHL/subscapularis tendon
  - The anterior structures are then inspected for tearing or fraying.
    - The rotator interval is seen, along with the upper portion of the tendon of the subscapularis.
    - The MGHL is seen traversing the subscapularis tendon.
    - The anterior band of the IGHL is seen inserting into the anteroinferior labrum.

- Rotator cuff
  - The arthroscope is brought superiorly, after looking at the biceps tendon, and the arm is then externally rotated and the camera is directed superiorly to inspect the rotator cuff near its insertion.

- The rotator cuff can be probed to detect partial thickness tears or other pathology.

- The supraspinatus tendon inserts at the articular margin of the superior humeral head.

- The arthroscope is gently retracted to evaluate the posterior rotator cuff insertion and bare area.

- Inferior labrum and axillary pouch

  - The camera is then moved inferiorly to inspect the axillary pouch, looking for loose bodies and evaluating the inferior labrum.

- Posterior labrum

  - The camera is then slowly withdrawn slightly while moving the lens proximally to evaluate the posterior labrum.

  - An attempt to elicit a "drive-through sign" can be made by moving the arthroscope between the glenoid and humeral head—usually only possible with laxity of the joint.

  - Alternatively, the arthroscopic camera can be inserted through the anterior cannula to assess the posterior labrum for a Bankart lesion or posterior partial thickness rotator cuff tears, as seen with internal impingement.

    ‣ The posterior portal is used for instrumentation when viewing anteriorly.

- Subacromial space

  - The camera is then placed in the posterior portal but directed more superiorly. The undersurface of the acromion is palpated with the trocar and sheath.

    ‣ The trochar is replaced by the camera.

    ‣ The bursa is inspected (may be swollen and erythematous with bursitis)

    ‣ The AC joint, acromion, and superior portion of the rotator cuff can also be assessed.

  - A lateral portal can be made for instrumentation. The portal is made using an outside-in technique and spinal needle for localization.

  - Radiofrequency devices or shavers can be used to aid in visualization of the space and structures.

    ‣ Because the bursa is quite vascular, regular shavers may cause bleeding which may affect visualization, and an electrocautery or radiofrequency device may be needed for hemostasis.

Common Arthroscopic Procedures

- Rotator cuff repair
  - The goal of rotator cuff repair, open or arthroscopic, is to reattach the avulsed tendon back to the humerus, restoring anatomy.
  - Arthroscopy has revolutionized the treatment of rotator cuff tears.
    - ▸ Arthroscopy has brought about a better understanding of rotator cuff tear patterns.
    - ▸ Arthroscopic rotator cuff repair and mini-open rotator cuff repair have nearly eliminated the risk of deltoid detachment.
    - ▸ Suture anchors and newer patterns of suture repair have helped improve strength of arthroscopic rotator cuff repair.
    - ▸ Special suture passers with flexible needles have been developed to pass sutures from anchors through the edge of the cuff (antegrade).
    - ▸ Sutures can also be passed with spinal needles or suture passers that are brought through portals and into the medial side of the rotator cuff (retrograde).
    - ▸ For U-shaped tears, side-to-side sutures can be placed through anterior and posterior portals (margin convergence) prior to repairing the lateral edge to the tuberosity, reducing the strain on the repair *(Fig. 5-5)*.

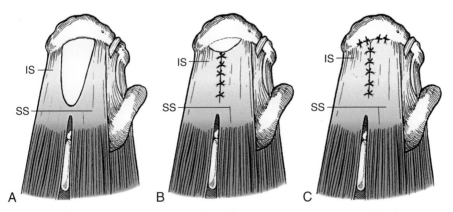

Figure 5-5. **A** through **C.** Margin convergence technique for repairing U-shaped tears of the rotator cuff. IS, infraspinatus; SS, supraspinatus. *(From Miller MD, Cole BJ. Textbook of Arthroscopy. Philadelphia, Elsevier, 2004 [Fig. 23-2, p 219].)*

- **SLAP (superior labral anterior to posterior) repairs**
  - Arthroscopy is responsible for the recognition, classification, and treament of SLAP tears.
  - These tears are classified into seven main types *(Fig. 5-6)*
  - Types I to IV were originally described. Types V to VII are associated with combined SLAP and labra tearing 360° lesions (triple labra tears; not pictured) were also been recognized.
  - Type II tears are the most common type of tear that requires arthroscopic treatment.

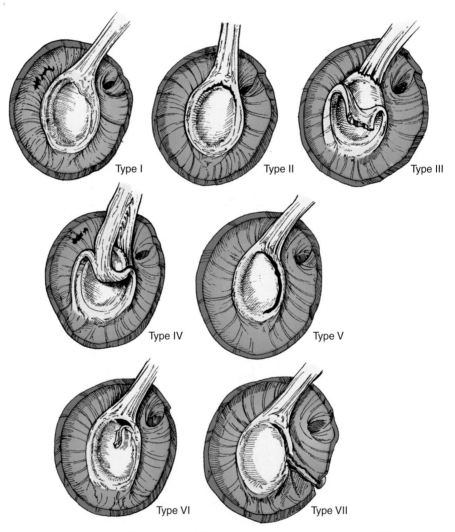

Figure 5-6. SLAP tear classification. *(From Miller MD, Osborne JR, Warner JJP, et al. MRI-Arthroscopy Correlative Atlas. Philadelphia, Saunders, 1997, p 157.)*

- Type II SLAP tears can be subclassified based on its location relation to the biceps origin:
  A. Anterior only
  B. Posterior only
  C. Anterior and posterior

- Typically, the superior glenoid is abraded, suture anchors are placed on both sides of the biceps, and sutures are passed and tied arthroscopically.

● Biceps tendon pathology

- Recognition of biceps tears has resulted in a marked increase in biceps tenotomies (release) and tenodesis (stabilization of the biceps and removal of the intra-articular portion).

- Biceps tendinopathy can be a "pain generator" as has been frequently recognized in patients with massive rotator cuff tears, and relief of pain after spontaneous biceps rupture.

- Arthroscopic release or tenodesis can result in significant pain relief.

- Tenodesis can be done with arthroscopic or open techniques and the tendon stump can be sutured to the rotator cuff or into a tunnel in the proximal humerus.

- Absorbable interference screws can be helpful to secure the tendon stump into a drill hole in the proximal humerus *(Fig. 5-7)*.

● Repair of labral tears

- In addition to superior labral tears, anterior and posterior labral tears can be fixed to the glenoid with suture anchors.

- Often these labral tears scar medially on the acetabular neck anterior labral periosteal sleeve avulsion (ALPSA) [Fig. 5-8] and must be mobilized—elevated up and onto the face of the glenoid prior to suture passage. One should see the muscle of the subscapularis to assure adequate elevation *(Fig. 5-8)*.

- The glenoid rim is abraded. Placing the anchor on the rim or medially will medialize the glenoid and not restore the bumper effect of the labrum. The labrum is placed partly onto the glenoid face, a few millimeters from the glenoid rim.

- Some capsular tightening or shift is usually also incorporated in the labral repair, because the plastic deformation of the capsule, if not addressed, may result in recurrent instability. Care is taken not to overtighten the capsule.

- Large cannulas assist in suture passage and knot-tying.

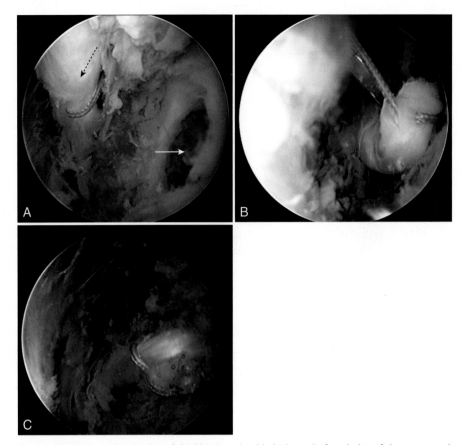

Figure 5-7. A. Anterosuperior view of the biceps tendon (*dashed arrow*) after placing of the sutures and drilling of the tunnel in the proximal humerus (*white arrow*). **B.** Free end of biceps tendon with suture being pushed into the blind-ended tenodesis tunnel. **C.** After biceps tenodesis is completed with tendon secured into the proximal tunnel. *(Courtesy of Anthony Romeo, MD.)*

- Acromioplasty and distal clavicle resection
  - An arthroscopic bursectomy is performed using a shaver with electocautery or with a radiofrequency ablation device to remove the bursa while providing the necessary hemostasis.

  - The coracoacromial ligament is cut with the electocautery or radiofrequency device to coagulate the acromial branch of the thoracoacromial artery. Confirmation that the ligament is cut all the way through when the muscular fibers of the deltoid can be seen from the subacromial space.

  - Care is taken to limit dissection medially because this is a vascular area.

  - An arthroscopic burr can be used to remove bone that impinges on the cuff or is a result of acromioclavicluar arthritis *(Fig. 5-9)*.

  - Bone removal may be performed by bringing the burr from the lateral portal and viewing from the posterior portal, which risks not removing enough bone medially.

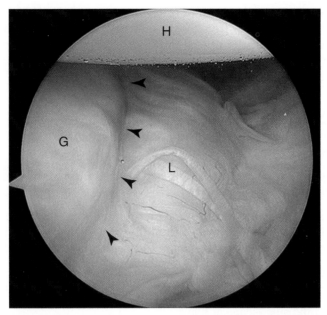

Figure 5-8. Anterior Labral Periosteal Sleeve Avulsion (ALPSA). ALPSA lesion (arrowheads). G, glenoid; H, humerus; L, labrum.

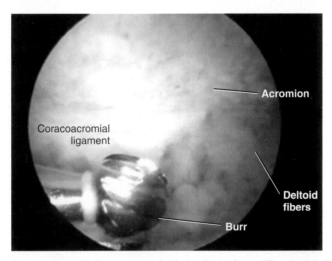

Figure 5-9. Using an arthroscopic burr to remove impinging bone. *(From Miller MD, Cole BJ. Textbook of Arthroscopy. Philadelphia, Elsevier, 2004 [Fig. 19-6, p 174].)*

- This may also be performed by bringing the burr from the posterior portal while viewing from the lateral portal, which risks leaving residual bone laterally.

- We encourage choosing one technique for the majority of the acromioplasty, but viewing from the other portal to confirm adequate decompression.

- Usually remove 2 to 4 mm of anterior acromion, and shaving the acromion so it is flat from back to front. This may be confirmed by placing the scope in the lateral portal and using a probe from the posterior portal to the anterior acromial edge to assure that the acromion is flat.

● **Adhesive capsulitis**

- This disease process may be global or may involve an area of the capsule such as the rotator interval (capsule between the subscapularis and biceps) or posteroinferior capsule.

- Manipulation under anesthesia may be attempted but often is combined with arthroscopic lysis of adhesions and/or capsulotomy.

- Care is taken when performing an arthroscopic capsulotomy, especially inferiorly, because the inferior capsule is within 1 cm, and in some cases may be in contact with, the axillary nerve.

- Arthroscopic shaving and ablation of this interval can be accomplished prior to manipulation under anesthesia *(Fig. 5-10).*

● **Release of the suprascapular nerve**

- Suprascapular nerve release has been performed arthroscopically with accessory portals to release the nerve at the transverse scapular ligament at the suprascapular notch as well as from the spinoglenoid notch and ligament.

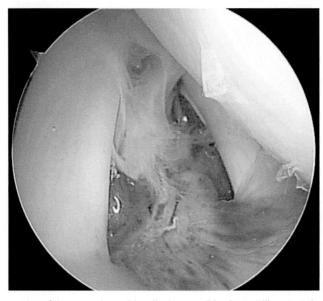

Figure 5-10. Scarring of the rotator interval in adhesive capsulitis. *(From Miller MD, Cole BJ. Textbook of Arthroscopy. Philadelphia, Elsevier, 2004 [Fig. 26-6, p 270].)*

Complications

- Neurovascular injury
  - Occurs most commonly when lateral decubitus position and traction are used. Some studies have reported from 10% to 30% incidence of traction palsies in this situation. It can be avoided by applying only 10 to 15 lbs of traction and positioning the arm in 45 to 70 degrees of abduction and 20 to 30 degrees of forward flexion. Be careful with padding the nonoperated arm as well as the peroneal nerve at the knee.
  - Placement of the anterior portal too medial and inferior also places neurovascular structures (cephalic vein and musculocutaneous nerve) at risk.
  - A lateral portal placed too distal or increasing the size of the lateral portal to convert to a mini-open rotator cuff repair may result in injury to the axillary nerve, which averages 6 cm from the lateral acromion.
  - Suprascapular nerve is 3-5 cm from the supraglenoid tubercle and may be at risk with extensive mobilization of a retracted rotator cuff tear, whereas the nerve is approximately 2 cm medial to the posterior border of the glenoid.
  - Ulnar nerve injury may occur to either arm when the patient is in the beach chair position.
  - The axillary nerve is also at risk when operating on the inferior capsule, because it may be adherent to the capsule and be injured during shoulder stabilization surgery or arthroscopic capsular release.
- Infection
  - Rare complication due to rich blood supply of the joint.
  - Most common organisms are *Staphylococcus epidermidis*, *Staphylococcus aureus*, and *Propionibacterium* species.
  - *Propionibacterium* species is an emerging cause of infection that has proved difficult to treat and may have a delayed presentation and may be hard to culture.
  - Often associated with destruction of the rotator cuff
- Deep vein thrombosis (DVT)
  - Very rare occurrence after shoulder arthroscopy
  - At this time, there is no indication for routine deep vein thrombosis (DVT) prophylaxis in patients unless they have risk factors such as a previous DVT/PE (pulmonary embolus) or known coagulopathies.

- Anesthesia complications
  - The use of regional anesthesia has its own inherent risks including neurovascular injury and pneumothorax if not performed properly.
  - Ultrasound guidance during the blocks may help reduce this risk.
- Arthrofibrosis
  - May occur after any procedure but unusual after simple arthroscopy
  - More likely to happen with concomitant rotator cuff and SLAP repair
- Iatrogenic chondromalacia
  - Seen more often after radiofrequency ablation of the capsule for instability.
  - Can be minimized with careful handling of radiofrequency devices
  - Careful use of instruments, especially with introduction of cannulas and trocars into the joint, can minimize risk.

REFERENCES

Baumfeld JA, Hart JA, and Miller MD. Sports Medicine. In Miller MD (ed). *Review of Orthopaedics*, 5th ed. Philadelphia, Saunders Elsevier, 2008.

Mazzocca AD, Alberta FG, Cole BJ, and Romeo AA. Shoulder: Patient positioning, portal placement, and normal arthroscopic anatomy. In Miller MD and Cole BJ (eds). *Textbook of Arthroscopy*, Philadelphia, Saunders, 2004.

Miller MD. Shoulder and arm. In Miller MD, Chhabra AB, and Hurwitz S, et al. (eds). *Orthopaedic Surgical Approaches*, Philadelphia, Saunders, 2008.

Miller MD, Howard RF, and Plancher KD. *Surgical Atlas of Sports Medicine*, Philadelphia, Saunders, 2003.

Shuler FD. Anatomy. In Miller MD (ed). *Review of Orthopaedics*, 5th ed., Philadelphia, Saunders Elsevier, 2008.

CHAPTER 6

ELBOW ARTHROSCOPY

Sara D. Rynders and A. Bobby Chhabra

Introduction

Elbow arthroscopy is a technically demanding procedure that may be used to evaluate and treat a variety of elbow disorders. Appropriate patient selection and knowledge of elbow anatomy, especially neurovascular anatomy, is critical to a good outcome.

Elbow arthroscopy was first described in the early 1930s, but did not become a viable operative technique until the 1980s, when arthroscopic equipment improved in quality and operative techniques became more refined. Since that time, elbow arthroscopy has evolved from a diagnostic tool to a treatment modality for multiple disorders of the elbow and its indications continue to expand.

- Indications
  - Limited elbow range of motion (ROM)
  - Mechanical symptoms of locking, popping, or catching
  - Mild-moderate osteoarthritis
  - Mayo grade 1 or 2 rheumatoid arthritis (RA)
  - Early post-traumatic arthritis with minimal deformity
  - Refractory lateral epicondylitis is a newer indication
  - Potential arthroscopic candidates should all have attempted and failed conservative measures such as therapy, NSAIDs, medical management of RA, activity modification and/or corticosteroid injections before proceeding to surgery.

- Common procedures performed include:
  - Diagnostic arthroscopy
  - Removal of loose bodies
  - Synovectomy
  - Osteophyte débridement
  - Capsular release
  - Ulnohumeral arthroplasty
  - Radial head resection
  - Lateral epicondyle débridement

- Arthroscopically assisted fracture reduction and fixation of certain simple fracture patterns

- Contraindications to elbow arthroscopy include:
  - The presence of significant heterotopic ossification

  - Local skin infection

  - The potential for noncompliance with postoperative therapy

  - Special consideration and relative contraindications include:
    ▸ Severe joint contractures

    ▸ Previous open elbow procedure or severe trauma resulting in distortion of the normal anatomic landmarks and joint surfaces

    ▸ Previous ulnar nerve transposition

    ▸ Displaced radial head or distal humerus fracture

Preoperative Considerations

- Preoperative workup
  - A thorough history and physical examination is essential. Document history of previous elbow injury, previous surgeries, presence of locking or instability, and the patient's current activity level and expectations.

  - Physical examination should include evaluation of elbow range of motion in all planes including supination and pronation and stress testing of the collateral ligaments. A thorough neurovascular examination should include evaluation of the ulnar nerve for the presence of cubital tunnel syndrome or subluxation of the nerve over the medial epicondyle with elbow flexion.

  - Appropriate elbow imaging may include radiographs with AP, lateral, and oblique views, MRI with or without arthrogram, CT scan, or diagnostic injections as indicated. If compressive neuropathy is suspected, EMG and nerve conduction studies are indicated.

  - Discuss realistic expectations of the surgical procedure and the anticipated recovery time.Therapy is usually indicated postoperatively to regain elbow ROM and this should be discussed with the patient in the preoperative setting.

- Anesthesia
  - General anesthesia is usually preferred. A regional intrascalene block is also an option but many surgeons opt for a postoperative block after the patient has had a thorough postoperative neurovascular examination.

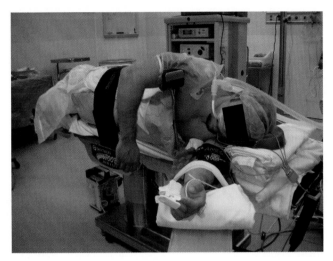

Figure 6-1. Patient position. Lateral decubitus position.

- Patient positioning *(Fig. 6-1)*
  - The patient may be placed supine, prone, or lateral decubitus depending on surgeon preference. This chapter will describe the lateral decubitus position. The patient is positioned on his or her side supported by a bean bag. The operative arm is placed on a padded arm holder with the shoulder at 90 degrees of forward flexion and the elbow is allowed to fall to gravity at 90 degrees. A nonsterile tourniquet (sterile may be used as well) is placed high on the brachium in the area supported by the arm holder to allow for maximal elbow ROM and access to the anterior elbow if necessary. The arm is then prepped and the patient is draped in a typical sterile manner. The monitor should be placed at the patient's back facing the arthroscopist. Gravity inflow should be used and pump inflow should be avoided because of the risks of compartment syndrome.

- Equipment
  - Padded arm holder
  - Sterile or nonsterile tourniquet
  - Arthroscope
  - Blunt trochar with cannula
  - 11 blade
  - Retractors
  - Shaver
  - Probe

- Graspers
- 18-gauge needle
- Lactated Ringer solution or Normal Saline suspended from IV pole
- Monitor and printer to document findings

Relevant Anatomy *(Fig. 6-2A-C)*

- Distal humerus
  - Capitellum
  - Trochlea
  - Coronoid fossa
  - Olecranon fossa
  - Lateral epicondyle
  - Medial epicondyle
  - Groove for ulnar nerve

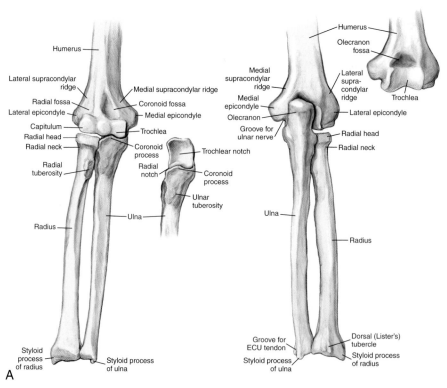

Figure 6-2. A. Elbow and forearm bony anatomy: volar view (*left*), dorsal view (*right*).

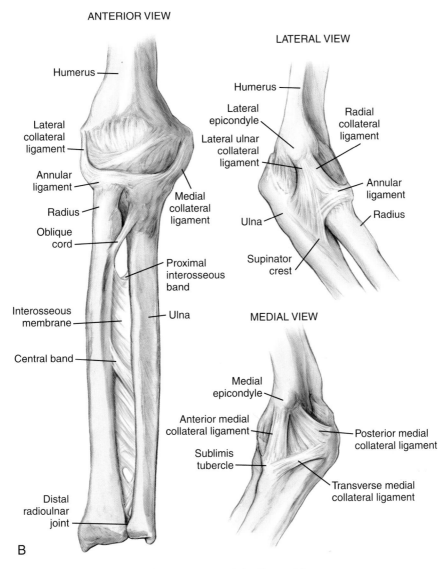

ANTERIOR VIEW

Humerus

Lateral
collateral
ligament

Annular
ligament

Radius

Oblique
cord

Medial
collateral
ligament

Proximal
interosseous
band

Interosseous
membrane

Ulna

Central band

Distal
radioulnar
joint

LATERAL VIEW

Humerus

Lateral
epicondyle

Lateral ulnar
collateral
ligament

Ulna

Radial
collateral
ligament

Annular
ligament

Radius

Supinator
crest

MEDIAL VIEW

Medial
epicondyle

Anterior medial
collateral ligament

Sublimis
tubercle

Posterior medial
collateral ligament

Transverse medial
collateral ligament

B

Figure 6-2—cont'd. B. Joint and ligament anatomy of the elbow and forearm.

(Continued)

- **Proximal radius**
  - Radial head
  - Radial neck
- **Proximal ulna**
  - Olecranon
  - Coronoid process

- Trochlear notch
- Radial notch for radial head at proximal radial-ulnar joint
- Ulnar collateral ligament
  - Anterior UCL
  - Posterior UCL
  - Transverse UCL
- Lateral collateral ligament complex
  - Lateral ulnar collateral ligament
  - Annular ligament
  - Radial collateral ligament
- Joint capsule

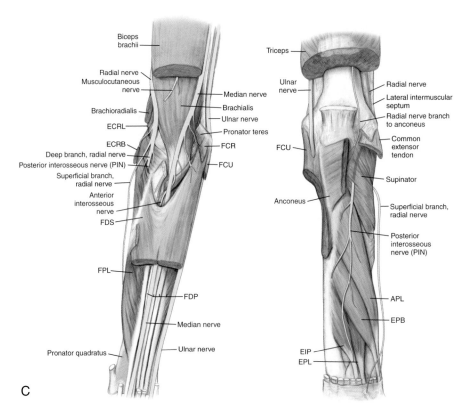

C

Figure 6-2—cont'd. **C.** Peripheral nerves at level of the elbow and volar forearm (*left*) and dorsal forearm (*right*). APL, abductor pollicis longus; ECRB, extensor carpi radialis brevis; ECRL, extensor carpi radialis longus; EIP, extensor indicis profundus; EPB, extensor pollicis brevis; EPL, extensor pollicis longus; FCR, flexor carpi radialis; FCU, flexor carpi ulnaris; FDP, flexor digitorum profundus; FDS, flexor digitorum superficialis; FPL, flexor pollicis longus. *(From Chhabra AB. Elbow and forearm. In Miller MD, Chhabra AB, Hurwitz S, et al. [eds]. Orthopaedic Surgical Approaches. Philadelphia, Elsevier, 2008, pp 63, 64, 67, 74, 75.)*

- Median nerve
  - Generally well protected because it crosses the elbow superficial to the large muscle belly of the brachialis
- Ulnar nerve
  - Crosses the elbow in the cubital tunnel, which lies directly superficial to the joint capsule in the medial gutter.
- Radial nerve and posterior interosseous nerve (PIN)
  - The radial nerve branches into a superficial sensory branch and a deep motor branch (PIN) just anterior to the lateral epicondyle.
  - The PIN crosses the elbow anterolaterally before piercing the supinator muscle and lies in close proximity to the anterolateral joint capsule.
- Cutaneous nerves
  - Medial antebrachial cutaneous
  - Posterior antebrachial cutaneous
  - Lateral antebrachial cutaneous
- Brachial artery

Portal Placement *(Fig. 6-3)*

- Anterior compartment
  - Anteromedial portal
    - May be one of the first portals established for introduction of the arthroscope.
    - Located 2 cm distal and 2 cm anterior to the medial epicondyle
    - Avoid injury to the anterior branch of the medial antebrachial cutaneous nerve during skin incision.
    - Used to visualize the capitellum, radial head, and anterior surface of the humerus
  - Proximal medial portal
    - Located 2 cm proximal to the medial epicondyle and just anterior to the medial intramuscular septum
    - Used to view the anterior compartment of the elbow and the lateral gutter. Many find it superior to the anteromedial portal.
    - This portal is in close proximity to the ulnar nerve, approximately 12 mm away, and is contraindicated in the setting of a subluxating ulnar nerve or a previous ulnar nerve transposition.

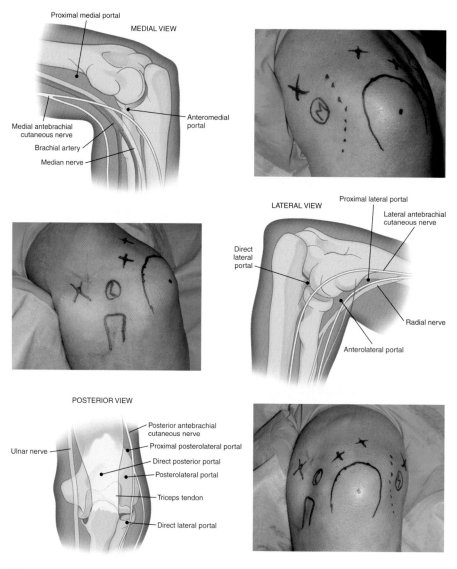

Figure 6-3. Portals. *(From Chhabra AB. Elbow and forearm. In Miller MD, Chhabra AB, Hurwitz S, et al. [eds]. Orthopaedic Surgical Approaches. Philadelphia, Elsevier, 2008, p 117.)*

▸ Avoid injury to the ulnar nerve during portal placement by aiming the trochar toward the radiocapitellar joint and sliding the trochar along the anterior aspect of the humerus.

▸ If a patient has a subluxating ulnar nerve, this portal should be made with extreme caution. When the ulnar nerve anatomy or location is variable, a mini-incision can be used to visualize the nerve and a retractor placed to protect the nerve before the portal is created.

- ▶ The medial antebrachial cutaneous nerve is at risk for injury because it lies approximately 2 mm from the portal.
- ■ Anterolateral portal
  - ▶ Located 3 cm distal and 1 cm anterior to the lateral epicondyle
  - ▶ Establish this portal with a spinal needle under direct visualization from the anteromedial portal.
  - ▶ Avoid injury to the anterior branch of the posterior antebrachial cutaneous nerve and the radial nerve, which should lie 2 to 10 mm anterior to the portal with the elbow in flexion.
- ■ Proximal lateral portal
  - ▶ Located 2 cm proximal and 1 cm anterior to the lateral epicondyle
  - ▶ Provides access to the anterior compartment. It may be preferred to the anterolateral portal because it is farther from the radial nerve (9 mm) and provides better visualization.
  - ▶ Avoid injury to the posterior branch of the lateral antebrachial cutaneous nerve located approximately 6 mm from the portal.
- ● **Posterior compartment**
  - ■ Posterolateral portal
    - ▶ Located at the level of the olecranon tip or 2 to 3 cm from the olecranon process, just lateral to the joint line with the elbow in 90 degrees of flexion.
    - ▶ Proximal and distal variations of this portal can be established in the same plane along the olecranon process.
    - ▶ Avoid injury to the medial and posterior antebrachial cutaneous nerves during portal placement.
    - ▶ Used to view the posterior compartment of the elbow including the olecranon tip, olecranon fossa, and posterior trochlea. This portal is also used to assess the medial gutter.
  - ■ Direct posterior portal
    - ▶ Located 3 cm proximal to the olecranon tip with the elbow in flexion and directly over the center of the triceps tendon.
    - ▶ The shaver can be placed into this portal without a cannula for débridement of the olecranon process and fossa under visualization from the posterolateral portal.

- Direct lateral portal (also known as midlateral portal)
  - Located in the "soft spot" between the lateral epicondyle, radial head, and olecranon process
  - Frequently used for joint insufflation
  - Avoid injury to the posterior antebrachial cutaneous nerve, which lies approximately 7 mm away.
  - This portal is used for visualization and débridement of the radiocapitellar joint.
- Posterior retractor portal
  - Located 2 cm proximal to the direct posterior portal
  - Used to introduce a retractor for better visualization or to elevate the posterior joint capsule

Diagnostic Arthroscopy (CPT 29830)

- Scope insertion
  - Arthroscopy begins with examination of the anterior compartment. Either the medial or lateral portals can be established first, based on preference.
  - Insufflate the elbow joint with 20 to 30 mL of normal saline at the soft spot located on the lateral aspect of the elbow, at the location of the midlateral portal site *(Fig. 6-4)*.

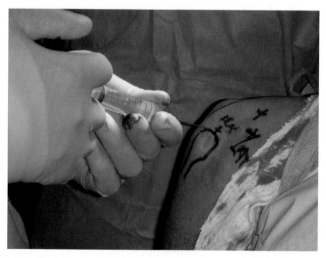

Figure 6-4. Joint insufflation.

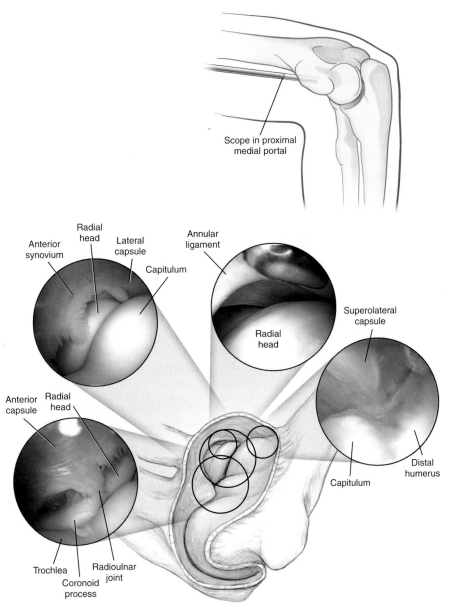

Figure 6-5. Proximal medial portal (anteromedial portal). *(From Chhabra AB. Elbow and forearm. In Miller MD, Chhabra AB, Hurwitz S, et al. [eds]. Orthopaedic Surgical Approaches. Philadelphia, Elsevier, 2008, p 119.)*

- ● **Anterior compartment**
  - ■ Proximal medial/anteromedial portal *(Fig. 6-5)*
    - ▸ Establish the proximal medial or anteromedial portal by making a small skin incision with an 11 blade. Use blunt

dissection to introduce the cannula and blunt obturator into the joint, followed by removal of the obturator and insertion of the arthroscope into the empty cannula. Gravity inflow of fluid should be used to maintain joint distention.

▸ Looking radially, identify the capitellum and radial head. It may be helpful to supinate/pronate the forearm to identify these structures.

▸ Moving ulnarly, identify the proximal radioulnar joint, coronoid process, and trochlea. The anterior joint capsule should also be in view.

▸ Pushing the scope more radially and distally, advance gently past the radial head to view the annular ligament.

▸ Looking radially and proximally, sliding the scope up along the capitellum, the superolateral capsule and lateral gutter is viewed.

- Proximal lateral/anterolateral portal *(Fig. 6-6)*

  ▸ With the arthroscope looking radially at the joint capsule just anterior to the capitellum, a spinal needle is inserted into the joint under direct visualization to establish the proximal lateral or anterolateral portal.

  ▸ Switch the arthroscope to this portal as soon as the cannula is established.

  ▸ Looking ulnarly now, identify the coronoid process and the trochlea. It may be helpful to place the elbow through flexion/extension ROM to identify these structures.

  ▸ The anterior joint capsule should also be viewed.

- **Posterior compartment**

  ▸ Maintain inflow anteriorly in the anterolateral or proximal lateral portal.

  - Posterolateral portal *(Fig. 6-7)*

    ▸ Establish this portal with an 11 blade and introduce the cannula with the blunt obturator into the posterior compartment of the joint. Aim the cannula ulnarly toward the olecranon tip, remove the obturator, and insert the arthroscope.

    ▸ View the lateral aspect of the olecranon and the posterior trochlea. It may help to place the elbow through flexion/extension ROM to identify these structures.

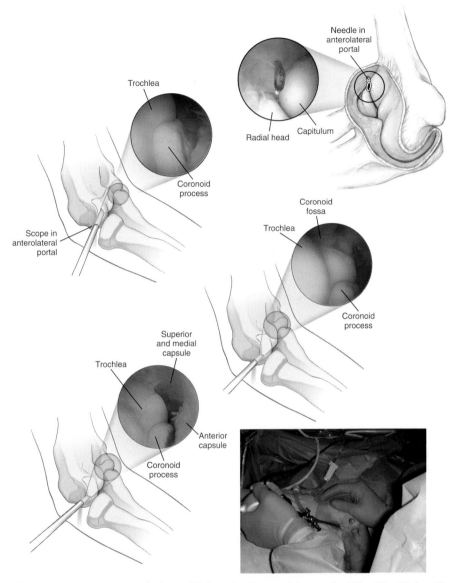

Figure 6-6. Anterolateral portal. *(From Chhabra AB. Elbow and forearm. In Miller MD, Chhabra AB, Hurwitz S, et al. [eds]. Orthopaedic Surgical Approaches. Philadelphia, Elsevier, 2008, pp 120-121.)*

■ Direct posterior portal *(Fig. 6-8)*

  ▶ This portal can be interchangeable as a viewing or working portal with the posterolateral portal.

  ▶ Position the arthroscope centrally and look down onto the olecranon tip. Examine the medial and lateral aspects of the olecranon process for impinging osteophytes.

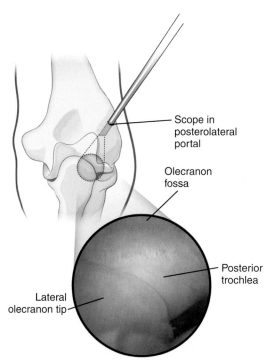

Figure 6-7. Posterolateral portal. *(From Chhabra AB. Elbow and forearm. In Miller MD, Chhabra AB, Hurwitz S, et al. [eds]. Orthopaedic Surgical Approaches. Philadelphia, Elsevier, 2008, p 123.)*

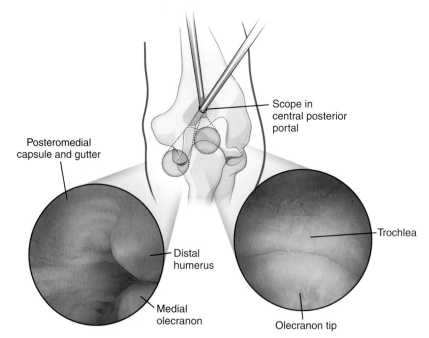

Figure 6-8. Direct posterior portal. *(From Chhabra AB. Elbow and forearm. In Miller MD, Chhabra AB, Hurwitz S, et al. [eds]. Orthopaedic Surgical Approaches. Philadelphia, Elsevier; 2008, p 123.)*

- With the elbow in flexion, the olecranon fossa can be viewed and débrided as necessary.

- Next, position the arthroscope to look ulnarly to evaluate the medial gutter. Place suction to gravity and USE EXTREME CAUTION in the medial gutter because the ulnar nerve lies directly superficial to the joint capsule. If use of a shaver is indicated for débridement, keep the blunt side of the shaver against the joint capsule at all times.

- Midlateral portal *(Fig. 6-9)*

  - This portal can be used for further evaluation of the lateral gutter.

  - Introduce the cannula with the blunt obturator, remove the obturator, and insert the arthroscope.

  - Aim the scope toward the olecranon process to view the lateral olecranon and the lateral aspect trochlear notch of the ulna.

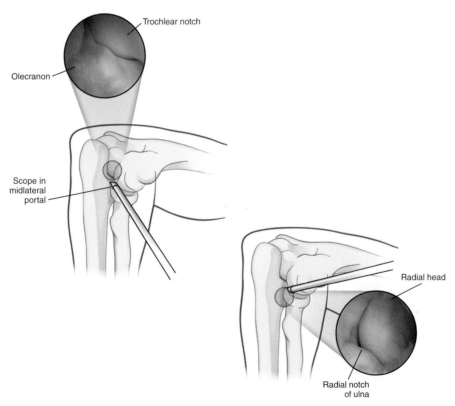

Figure 6-9. Midlateral portal. *(From Chhabra AB. Elbow and forearm. In Miller MD, Chhabra AB, Hurwitz S, et al. [eds]. Orthopaedic Surgical Approaches. Philadelphia, Elsevier, 2008, p 122.)*

▸ Next, position the arthroscope downward to view distally and examine the lateral aspect of the radial head and the dorsal aspect of the proximal radioulnar joint.

Common Arthroscopic Procedures

Synovectomy, Débridement, and Removal of Loose Bodies (CPT: Loose Bodies 29834, Synovectomy Partial/Complete 29835/29836, Débridement Limited/Extensive 29837/29838) *(Fig. 6-10)*

Synovectomy may be partial or complete and is most commonly performed in patients with rheumatoid arthritis. Arthroscopic synovectomy has been found to be most reliable in Mayo grade 1 or 2 rheumatoid disease with an earlier reported return to function than with an open procedure. Osteophyte débridement and removal of loose bodies is usually indicated in the osteoarthritic or early post-traumatic elbow. Débridement is performed with a shaver and large loose bodies are removed with a grasper. Pay special attention to the coronoid fossa, olecranon fossa, and olecranon tip as osteophytes and loose bodies are commonly found in these areas and elbow ROM can be significantly improved simply by their removal or débridement.

The surgeon should be comfortable with switching portals to maximize access to the joint while at the same time protecting all neurovascular structures. Mini-incisions and placement of retractors to protect certain neurovascular structures is often helpful and improves safety.

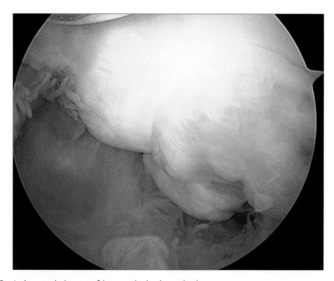

Figure 6-10. Arthroscopic image of intra-articular loose body.

Capsule Release (CPT 24006-52)

An anterior capsule release is performed to improve elbow extension; a posterior capsule release is performed to improve elbow flexion. A periosteal elevator is introduced into the joint to elevate the capsule and release adhesions. A capsulotomy can also be performed with use of a duckbill basket biopsy punch or similar cutting instrument. The capsule is incised from medial to lateral along its midsection with care taken to avoid injury to the anterior neurovascular structures which are protected by the brachialis muscle belly. The shaver should be kept facing the distal humerus and not turned anteriorly during anterior capsular release to prevent injury to the anterior neurovascular structures. When performing a posterior capsule release, pay close attention while working near the medial gutter to avoid injury to the ulnar nerve. A retractor can be placed to protect the ulnar nerve if necessary.

Radial Head Excision (CPT 24130-52)

This procedure is generally performed in conjunction with synovectomy in the rheumatoid patient who complains of painful and restricted forearm rotation due to impingement at the proximal radioulnar joint. This procedure was more widely used in the 1980s and now seems to be falling out of favor with development of better radial head implants and total elbow prostheses. Radial head excision is performed using the proximal medial, anterolateral, and direct lateral portals. The arthroscope is placed into the proximal medial portal to visualize the radial head and a burr is placed through the working anterolateral portal. The burr is used very carefully to expose trabecular bone. When accomplished, a shaver is placed into the anterolateral portal and the anterior three quarters of the radial head and 2 to 3 mm of the radial neck are carefully resected. Intraoperative fluoroscopy should be available and used periodically during this procedure to avoid over-resection. Structures at risk during this procedure include the PIN, which overlies the anterolateral joint capsule and the annular ligament. When the anterior portion of the radial head and neck is excised, an abrader is introduced into the direct lateral portal and the remainder of the posterior radial head and neck are removed.

Ulnohumeral Arthroplasty (CPT 24140-52) *(Fig. 6-11)*

Ulnohumeral arthroplasty can be a technically demanding procedure when placed under the time constraints necessary for arthroscopy. The procedure begins after the posterior compartment has been débrided. A 5-mm drill bit is used to drill a hole through the center of the olecranon fossa through the humerus to the center of the coronoid fossa anteriorly. Next, a notch-plasty blade or burr is used to widen the hole until full flexion of ≥135 degrees and full extension of 0 to −5 degrees is attained. Often complete fenestration of the humerus is unnecessary to improve ROM, and simple débridement, widening,

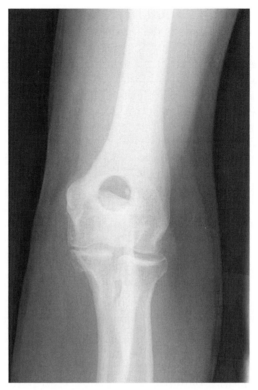

Figure 6-11. Postoperative radiograph. Ulnohumeral arthroplasty with complete fenestration of the distal humerus. *(From Rynders SR, Manke C. Arthroscopic treatment of the arthritic elbow. In Arthritis and Arthroplasty. Philadelphia, Elsevier, 2009, p 212.)*

and deepening the olecranon fossa is sufficient. When complete fenestration is performed, the hole should be enlarged no further than the medial and lateral humeral columns and its width should be monitored by intermittent use of intraoperative fluoroscopy. Arthroscopy of the anterior compartment should be performed as well to remove any anterior osteophytes or loose bodies.

Lateral Epicondyle Débridement (See Débridement Limited/ Extensive CPT 29837/29838)

Arthroscopic lateral epicondyle débridement is an emerging alternative to the traditional open débridement procedure. The anteromedial or proximal medial portal is used as the viewing portal and the proximal lateral portal is used as the working portal. There is a *safe zone* with this procedure located between the anterior half of the radial head with the elbow in flexion and the distal border of the extensor carpi radialis longus (ECRL) tendon insertion *(Fig. 6-12)*. Working within this safe zone minimizes the risk of injury to either the posterior interosseous nerve (PIN) or the lateral collateral ligament (LCL). First the proximal portion of the extensor carpi radialis brevis (ECRB) tendon is released

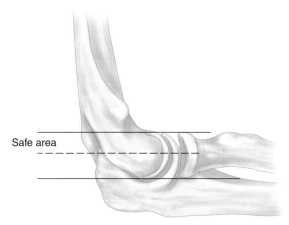

Figure 6-12. Lateral epicondyle débridement "safe zone." (Redrawn from Calfee RP, Patel A, DaSilva MF, Akelman E. Management of lateral epicondylitis: Current concepts. J Am Acad Orthop Surg 2008;16:19-29.)

from the lateral epicondyle and lateral condylar ridge. The lateral epicondyle is then decorticated with a burr or shaver with care taken to avoid injury to the articular surface.

Arthroscopic-assisted Fracture Reduction

- **Capitellum fractures (CPT 24579-52)**
  - Capitellum fractures, while rare, require adequate reduction to restore the radiocapitellar articular surface and the stability provided by the lateral column. An arthroscopic technique (versus a traditional open procedure) has been described for minimally displaced fractures (type I or II) to limit elbow stiffness and provide better visualization for accurate fracture reduction, thus reducing the risk for post-traumatic arthritis. The anterolateral portal is used for instrumentation and the proximal lateral portal is used for viewing. Additional portals may be used as indicated to reduce the fracture fragment. When the fracture is manipulated into a reduced position, K wires are placed to hold the reduction. Cannulated screws are then driven over the wires and buried subchondrally. Intraoperative fluoroscopy should be used frequently to confirm adequate reduction.

- **Radial head fractures (CPT 24665-52)**
  - Open reduction and internal fixation is still the gold standard of treatment for displaced radial head fractures. However, arthroscopic fracture reduction and percutaneous fixation has been implicated in the management of minimally displaced Mason type II-III fractures and in patients with nondisplaced fractures and continued pain. The proximal medial portal is

used for viewing and the proximal lateral portal is used for instrumentation. First, the anterior compartment is débrided for better visualization and the articular cartilage is evaluated. The fracture is visualized and a Kirschner wire is placed through the anterolateral portal into the fracture fragment to act as a joystick during reduction. When reduced, the wire is driven across the fracture and a cannulated screw is driven over the wire. Intraoperative fluoroscopy is used judiciously to assess reduction. When reduced, and if additional fixation is deemed necessary, attention is turned toward the posterolateral aspect of the joint. The direct lateral portal is established as a viewing portal and the posterolateral portal is established as a working portal (or any area 1 to 2 cm proximal to the direct lateral portal along the border of the olecranon and triceps tendon). The posterolateral elbow joint is débrided and the fracture is identified. Again a guidewire is placed across the fracture and a cannulated screw is placed over the wire. The posterior compartment of the elbow should be thoroughly débrided before closure. Arthroscopic-assisted fracture reduction is challenging and should be performed only by the experienced elbow arthroscopist.

Complications

- Nerve injury
  - There is a higher risk of nerve injury in arthroscopy of the elbow than arthroscopy of any other major joints.
  - Transient neurapraxia is the most commonly reported complication of elbow arthroscopy.
  - There is increased incidence of transient neurapraxia in patients with a preoperative elbow contracture or an underlying diagnosis of rheumatoid arthritis.
  - Cutaneous nerve injury can occur during portal placement and can be minimized by blunt dissection to the joint capsule and use of a blunt obturator during cannulization.
  - The most common neurapraxic injury occurs to the ulnar nerve due to its close proximity to the medial gutter. Care should be taken while working in this area to keep shavers pointed AWAY from the joint capsule. Also, the proximal medial portal should NEVER be used in the setting of a transposed or subluxating ulnar nerve.

- ■ The most common major motor nerve injury occurs to the radial nerve or PIN as it crosses the anterolateral elbow. Risk of injury is minimized by meticulous work near the anterolateral joint capsule with care taken to avoid compromise. Supinating the forearm while working in this area can aid in pushing the PIN farther from the joint capsule.

- ■ It is imperative that a surgeon perform and document an immediate postoperative neurovascular examination before any regional anesthesia is administered.

- ● Septic joint
  - ■ Minimize this risk with good sterile technique, appropriately sterilized instruments, and use of preoperative intravenous antibiotics.

- ● Portal fistulas
  - ■ Meticulous wound closure with suture will generally prevent this complication. Use of postoperative drains increases the risk of fistula formation.

- ● Elbow stiffness
  - ■ Loss of 30 degrees or less of elbow motion is considered a minor complication.

  - ■ Minimize this risk by appropriate postoperative edema control, adequate pain control, and initiation of early ROM within the first 3 to 5 postoperative days.

  - ■ Some surgeons advocate static progressive splinting or continuous passive motion (CPM) in the immediate postoperative period but evidence to support these measures is inconclusive.

- ● Compartment syndrome
  - ■ Extravasation of fluid from the elbow joint can cause arm or forearm compartment syndrome.

  - ■ The risk of this complication is minimized by limiting the number of times the elbow capsule is violated, by working efficiently to decrease the duration of the procedure, by close intraoperative monitoring of the soft tissues for increased turgor, and by the use of gravity fluid inflow.

- ● Hemarthrosis
  - ■ Some surgeons advocate the use of a Hemovac drain and 36 hours of elevation in an extension splint; others feel that a standard postoperative compression dressing and elevation is sufficient.

REFERENCES

Andrews J and Carson W. Arthroscopy of the elbow. *Arthroscopy* 1985; 1:97–107.

Baker CL and Jones GL. Arthroscopy of the elbow. *Am J Sports Med* 1999; 27:251–264.

Baker CL, Murphy KP, Gottlob CA, and Curd DT. Arthroscopic classification and treatment of lateral epicondylitis: Two year clinical results. *J Shoulder Elbow Surg* 2000; 9(6):475–482.

Calfee RP, Patel A, DaSilva MF, and Akelman E. Management of lateral epicondylitis: Current concepts. *J Am Acad Orthop Surg* 2008; 16:19–29.

Chhabra AB. Elbow and forearm. In Miller MD, Chhabra AB, and Hurwitz S, et al. (eds). *Orthopaedic Surgical Approaches*, Philadelphia, Elsevier, 2008; pp 115–125.

Dodson CC, Nho SJ, Williams RJ, and Altcheck DW. Elbow arthroscopy. *J Am Acad Orthop Surg* 2008; 16(10):574–585.

Geissler WB. Arthroscopic assisted fixation of radial head fractures. In Trumble TE and Budoff FE (eds). *Wrist and Elbow Reconstruction & Arthroscopy*, Rosemont, Ill, ASSH, 2006; pp 479–488.

Hardy P, Menguy F, and Guillot S. Arthroscopic treatment of capitellum fracture of the humerus. *Arthroscopy—J Orthop Rel Surg* 2002; 18(4):422–426.

Hsu J and Yamaguchi K. Elbow: anesthesia, patient positioning, portal placement, normal arthroscopic anatomy, and diagnostic arthroscopy. In Miller MD and Cole BI (eds). *Textbook of Arthroscopy*, Philadelphia, Elsevier, 2004; pp 289–306.

Kelly EW, Morrey BF, and O'Driscoll SW. Complications of elbow arthroscopy. *J Bone Joint Sur* 2001; 83(1):25–34.

Menth-Chiari WA, Poehling GG, and Ruch DS. Arthroscopic resection of the radial head. *Arthroscopy—J Arthros Rel Sur* 1999; 15(2):226–230.

Miller D, Gregory JJ, and Hay SM. Arthroscopy of the elbow. *Curr Orthop* 2008; 22(2):104–110.

Rosenburg B and Loebenberg M. Elbow arthroscopy. *Bull NYU Hosp Jt Dis* 2007; 56(1):43–50.

Savoie FH, Nunley PD, and Field LD. arthroscopic management of the arthritic elbow: Indications, technique, and results. *J Shoulder Elbow Surg* 1999; 8(3): 214–219.

Steinmann SP. Elbow arthroscopy: Where are we now? *Arthroscopy—the Journal of Arthroscopic and Related Surgery* 2007; 23(11):1231–1236.

Strothers K, Day B, and Regan WR. Arthroscopy of the elbow—anatomy, portal sites, and a description of the proximal lateral portal. *Arthroscopy* 1995; 11(4):449–457.

WRIST ARTHROSCOPY

Sara D. Rynders and A. Bobby Chhabra

Introduction

Arthroscopy of the wrist is commonly used for the evaluation and treatment of multiple wrist disorders including chronic wrist pain, interosseous ligament tears, triangular fibrocartilage complex tears, ganglion cysts, and wrist synovitis. Arthroscopy is considered the gold standard for the diagnosis of intra-articular ligamentous injuries and is becoming more widely used as a visual aid during intra-articular fracture reduction and fixation and shortening osteotomies. A detailed understanding of wrist anatomy and biomechanics is essential to successful arthroscopy.

- Indications
  - Diagnosis of wrist pain
  - Synovitis and loose bodies
  - Known or suspected scapholunate ligament (SLL) or lunotriquetral ligament (LTL) tears
  - Triangular fibrocartilage complex (TFCC) tears
  - Ganglion cysts
  - Intra-articular distal radius fractures
  - Scaphoid fractures
  - Ulnocarpal impaction
- Common procedures performed
  - Diagnostic arthroscopy
  - Synovectomy, débridement, and removal of loose bodies
  - TFC débridement or repair
  - SLL or LTL repair or débridement
  - Arthroscopic ganglionectomy
  - Arthroscopically assisted distal radius and scaphoid fracture reduction
  - Ulnar-shortening osteotomy

- Contraindications to wrist arthroscopy include
  - Local skin infection
  - Previous injury with significant scarring or derangement of normal anatomic landmarks
  - Moderate-to-severe wrist arthritis preventing insertion of arthroscope

Preoperative Considerations

- Preoperative workup
  - A thorough history and physical examination of the wrist should be performed prior to surgery and preoperative wrist range of motion, grip strength, and a detailed neurovascular examination should be noted.
  - Imaging modalities such as radiographs, MRI, CT, ultrasound, or fluoroscopic arthrogram should be used as indicated to aid in diagnosis.
  - Selective diagnostic intra-articular injections may be used as a preoperative diagnostic modality.
  - The patient should be counseled on the anticipated outcome or goal of the surgery, including the risks and benefits and the expected course of recovery.
  - If a diagnostic arthroscopy is planned, the patient should give consent for any procedures that may be indicated by the intra-operative findings and should be made aware of the expected postoperative course, given each situation.
- Anesthesia
  - Local, general, or regional anesthesia or any combination thereof
  - A regional block such as an intrascalene or supraclavicular block preoperatively with administration of general anesthesia is usually preferred.
- Patient positioning *(Fig. 7-1)*
  - Patient is placed supine on the operating table with the operative upper extremity extended onto an armboard at the patient's shoulder level.
  - A nonsterile tourniquet is applied to the patient's brachium but not inflated, or a sterile tourniquet may be applied later in the surgery if conversion to an open procedure is planned or deemed necessary by arthroscopic findings.

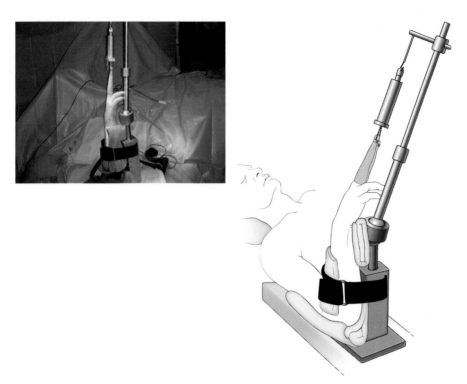

Figure 7-1. Patient positioning. *(From Chhabra AB. Wrist and hand. In Miller MD, Chhabra AB, Hurwitz S, et al. [eds]. Orthopaedic Surgical Approaches. Philadelphia, Elsevier, 2008; p 188.)*

- The patient is prepped and draped using standard technique.

- The surgeon stands at the patient's head facing the dorsal aspect of the wrist and the patient's feet. The monitor is set up at the patient's feet facing the surgeon.

- The Mayo tray is placed on the armboard under the patient's operative arm to provide a stable base.

- The traction tower is placed on the Mayo stand. The patient's elbow is flexed to 90 degrees in neutral pronation. The volar aspect of the patient's forearm should lie against the traction tower. Padding is applied as indicated.

- Two straps are used to secure the arm to the tower: one strap wraps under the Mayo stand and secures the patient's brachium; the other strap secures the traction tower to the patient's forearm.

- 30 degrees of volar tilt is applied to the traction tower to place the wrist into a slightly flexed position.

- The tower is fitted with the traction gauge and the finger traps are applied (tip: if patient's fingers slide out of the traps, a self-adhesive bandage or tape can be wrapped around the finger before applying the trap to prevent slipping). Typically the index and middle fingers are suspended for traction, but if particular attention is going to be paid to the ulnar side of the wrist, the ulnar fingers may be suspended also.

- The tower is adjusted to provide 15 lb of traction force across the wrist.

● Equipment
- Armboard attached to operating table.
- Mayo tray
- Traction tower
- Traction gauge
- Towels for padding
- Straps
- Finger traps
- Arthroscope
- Monitor and printer to document findings
- Probe
- Blunt trochar
- Shaver
- Set of arthroscopic graspers and biters
- 18-Gauge needle for outflow
- Lactated Ringer solution or Normal Saline suspended from IV pole

Relevant Anatomy

● Extensor tendon compartments *(Fig. 7-2)*
- 1st: extensor pollicis brevis, abductor pollicis longus (EPB, APL)
- 2nd: extensor carpi radialis brevis, extensor carpi radialis longus (ECRB, ECRL)
- 3rd: extensor pollicis longus (EPL)
- 4th: extensor digitorum communis, extensor indicis proprius (EDC, EIP)
- 5th: extensor digiti minimi (EDM)
- 6th: extensor carpi ulnaris (ECU)

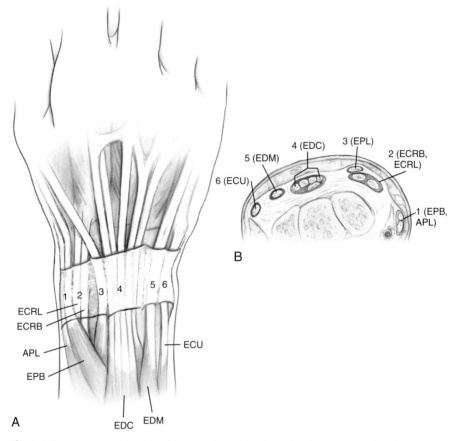

Figure 7-2. Extensor compartments. *(From Chhabra AB. Wrist and hand. In Miller MD, Chhabra AB, Hurwitz S, et al. [eds]. Orthopaedic Surgical Approaches. Philadelphia, Elsevier, 2008; p 156.)*

- Radiocarpal joint *(Fig. 7-3)*
  - Radius with scaphoid and lunate fossae
  - Ulna and ulnar styloid
  - Prestyloid recess
  - Distal radioulnar joint and sigmoid notch
  - Proximal carpal row: scaphoid, lunate, triquetrum (pisiform)
  - The TFCC is located on the ulnar aspect of the wrist and stabilizes the distal radiioulnar joint (DRUJ). It is poorly vascularized centrally but has adequate peripheral blood flow. It is composed of
    - Fibrocartilage disc
    - Volar and dorsal distal radioulnar ligaments

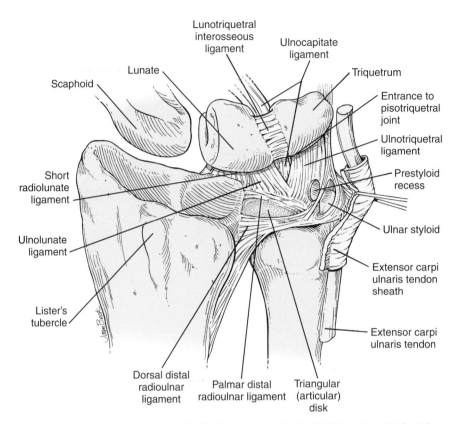

Figure 7-3. Radiocarpal joint anatomy. *(Modified from Cooney WP, Linscheid RL, Dobyns JH. The Wrist: Diagnosis and Operative Treatment. St. Louis, C.V. Mosby, 1998.)*

- ‣ Meniscus homolog

- ‣ Volar ulnocarpal ligaments: ulnolunate and ulnotriquetral ligaments

- ‣ ECU tendon sub sheath

- Mid-carpal joint

   - Distal carpal row: trapezium, trapezoid, capitate, hamate.

   - Can visualize the distal scaphoid, lunate, and triquetrum of the proximal row

- Ligaments *(Fig. 7-4)*

   - Interosseous

      - ‣ Scapholuate ligament (SLL): C-shaped ligament which is thinner and weaker volarly and stronger and thicker dorsally.

      - ‣ Lunotriquetral ligament (LTL)

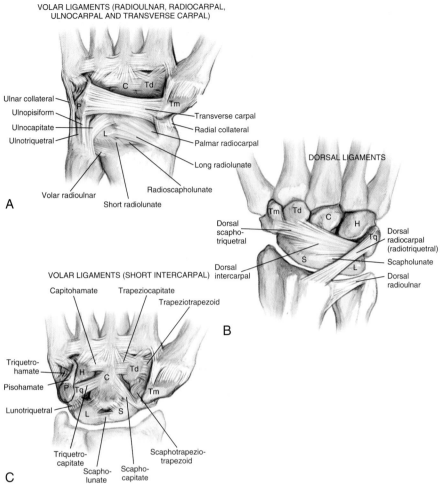

VOLAR LIGAMENTS (RADIOULNAR, RADIOCARPAL, ULNOCARPAL AND TRANSVERSE CARPAL)

Ulnar collateral
Ulnopisiform
Ulnocapitate
Ulnotriquetral

Transverse carpal
Radial collateral
Palmar radiocarpal
Long radiolunate
Radioscapholunate

Volar radioulnar
Short radiolunate

A

DORSAL LIGAMENTS

Dorsal scapho-triquetral
Dorsal intercarpal

Dorsal radiocarpal (radiotriquetral)
Scapholunate
Dorsal radioulnar

B

VOLAR LIGAMENTS (SHORT INTERCARPAL)

Capitohamate
Trapeziocapitate
Trapeziotrapezoid

Triquetro-hamate
Pisohamate
Lunotriquetral

Triquetro-capitate
Scapho-lunate
Scapho-capitate
Scaphotrapezio-trapezoid

C

Figure 7-4. Ligaments. *(From Chhabra AB. Wrist and hand. In Miller MD, Chhabra AB, Hurwitz S, et al [eds]. Orthopaedic Surgical Approaches. Philadelphia, Elsevier, 2008; p 150.)*

- Extrinsic ligaments:
  ▸ Radioscaphoid ligament (RS)
  ▸ Radioscaphocapitate ligament (RSC)
  ▸ Long and short radiolunate ligaments (LRL, SRL)
  ▸ Radioscapholunate ligament (RSL, also known as ligament of Testut—contains neurovascular supply to the SLL and lunate; sometimes not considered a ligament because it is often found within loose connective tissue)
  ▸ Ulnolunate and ulnotriquetral ligaments (part of TFCC)
  ▸ Dorsal intercarpal ligament
  ▸ Dorsal radiocarpal ligament

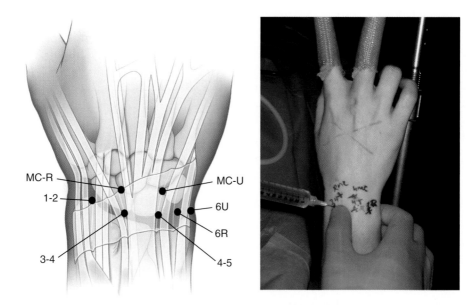

Figure 7-5. Portals. *(From Chhabra AB. Wrist and hand. In Miller MD, Chhabra AB, Hurwitz S, et al [eds]. Orthopaedic Surgical Approaches. Philadelphia, Elsevier, 2008; p 189.)*

Portal Placement *(Fig. 7-5)*

- All portals are named based on the bordering extensor compartments and are located such that important neurovascular and tendinous structures are protected. Although there are 12 portals that may be used, the most common portals are the 1-2, 3-4, 4-5, mid-carpal radial (MC-R), and mid-carpal ulnar (MC-U), 6U and 6R.

  - 3-4 portal

    ▸ Between the 3rd and 4th extensor compartments approximately 1 cm distal and ulnar to Lister's tubercle in the "soft spot" of the radiocarpal joint.

    ▸ This is the first portal to be established for most procedures and is used for introduction of the arthroscope into the radiocarpal joint.

  - 4-5 portal

    ▸ Between the 4th and 5th extensor compartments at the level of the radiocarpal joint.

    ▸ Establish this portal under visualization from the 3-4 portal.

    ▸ This is the first instrument portal.

- 6R portal

  ▸ Radial to the 6th extensor compartment between the EDM and ECU tendons at the level of the radiocarpal joint

  ▸ Establish under direct visualization from the 3-4 portal.

  ▸ Used for TFCC repairs.

- 6U portal

  ▸ Ulnar (or volar) to the 6th extensor compartment

  ▸ Used for TFCC repairs

  ▸ Take caution to avoid injury to dorsal sensory branch of ulnar nerve

- 1-2 portal

  ▸ Between the 1st and 2nd extensor compartments and radial to the 3rd extensor compartment

  ▸ Take caution to avoid injury to the radial artery in the anatomical snuffbox

- Midcarpal radial portal

  ▸ Approximately 1 cm distal to the 3-4 portal, bordered by the ECRB and the 4th extensor compartment at the level of the mid-carpal joint.

  ▸ Used as arthroscope portal for evaluation of the mid-carpal joint, scapholunate ligament, and lunotriquetral ligament.

- Mid-carpal ulnar portal

  ▸ Approximately 1 cm distal to the 4-5 portal between the 4th and 5th extensor compartments at the level of the mid-carpal joint

  ▸ Used as instrument portal when evaluating structures of the mid-carpal joint

- Other portals

  ▸ Distal radioulnar joint portal

    • Working portal: Located just proximal to the DRUJ and the 4-5 working portal, bordered by the radius and ulna and the 4th and 5th extensor compartments

    • Viewing portal: located more proximal than the working portal just ulnar to the 5th extensor compartment.

  ▸ Scaphoid-trapezium-trapezoid portal

- Located just ulnar to the 3rd extensor compartment and just radial of the ECRB insertion at the level of the distal pole of the scaphoid.

  ▸ Triquetrohamate portal

- Located just distal to the 6U portal between the insertion point of the ECU and the EDM at the level of the mid-carpal joint

  ▸ Volar radial (VR) portal

- A 2-cm longitudinal incision is made over the flexor carpi radialis (FCR) tendon. FCR is identified and retracted ulnarly.

- A needle is used to establish this portal under direct visualization from the 3-4 portal.

  ▸ Volar ulnar (VU) portal

- A 2-cm longitudinal incision is made over the FCU. FCU is identified and retracted ulnarly, thereby protecting the ulnar nerve.

- Develop an interval between the FCU and common flexor tendons.

- A needle is used to establish this portal under direct visualization from the 3-4 or 4-5 portal.

Diagnostic Arthroscopy (CPT 29840)

- Joint insufflation
  - 10 mL of normal saline is injected into the radiocarpal joint at the 3-4 portal for joint distention.
  - If a tourniquet is being used, it may be inflated at this time.

- Scope insertion *(Fig. 7-6)*
  - The 3-4 portal is marked and a small skin incision is made with an 11 blade parallel to the extensor tendons.
  - The scope cannula containing the blunt trochar is inserted into the incision. The trochar is removed, and the arthroscope is introduced into the radiocarpal joint.
  - Gravity inflow is connected to the arthroscope and an outflow needle is placed at the 6R portal under visualization to clear the visual field.
  - Orient the camera's visual field so that the distal radius is at the bottom of the monitor screen, the proximal row at the top.

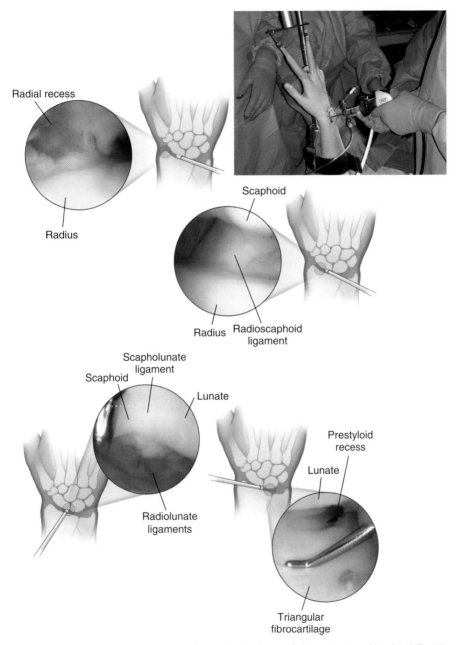

Figure 7-6. Diagnostic arthroscopy of the radiocarpal joint. *(From Chhabra AB. Wrist and hand. In Miller MD, Chhabra AB, Hurwitz S, et al. [eds]. Orthopaedic Surgical Approaches. Philadelphia, Elsevier, 2008; p 191.)*

- The 4-5 portal may be established in the same way as the 3-4 portal at this point, while under direct visualization from the 3-4 portal. Probes, shavers, or graspers may be introduced through this portal as necessary.

- **Distal radius, radial styloid, and radial recess**
  - The lens is rotated radially to begin the evaluation.
  - The surface of the distal radius and the scaphoid fossa are identified. The scope is introduced further into the joint and slid up the surface of the radius to visualize the radial styloid and just beyond, the radial recess in the joint capsule.
  - Inspect for osteophytes, osteochondral lesions, synovitis, or disruption of the capsule.
- **Proximal scaphoid**
  - As the lens is rotated back to neutral and the scope is oriented volarly, the proximal surface of the scaphoid is examined for occult proximal pole fractures or chondral lesions.
- **Radioscaphocapitate, long and short radiolunate ligaments**
  - Visualized directly volar to the 3-4 portal. The radioscaphocapitate ligament is radial to the long and short radiolunate ligaments. Evaluate for synovitis or ligament fraying.
- **Scapholunate ligament**
  - With the arthroscope oriented volarly the lens is rotated in an upward direction to identify the SLL. Evaluate the ligament for fraying which can raise suspicion for a tear.
- **Proximal lunate and lunate fossa**
  - Identify the lunate adjacent to the scaphoid and evaluate for chondral lesions which could indicate evidence of ulnocarpal impaction. Orient the lens to look in a downward fashion onto the distal radius surface and the lunate fossa. Assess for chondral lesions.
- **TFCC**
  - Looking ulnarly from the lunate fossa, the triangular fibrocartilage of the TFCC is identified overlying the distal ulna and connecting to the ulnar aspect of the distal radius. Assess the entire surface of the triangular fibrocartilage looking for defects, fraying, perforations, or degenerative tearing.
  - Insert a probe through the 4-5 portal and perform a trampoline test—the probe should rebound from the fibrocartilage disk if it is healthy and intact. Lack of rebound may indicate degenerative thinning or raise suspicion for a tear (*Fig. 7-7*).
  - If a tear is identified, its location and severity (incomplete versus complete) should be documented.

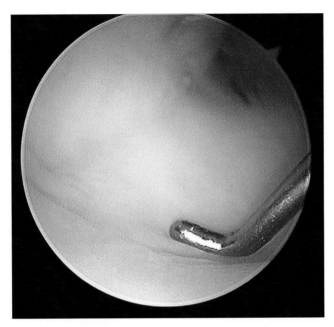

Figure 7-7. Trampoline test of the TFCC.

- Slide the arthroscope ulnarly to view the ulnar gutter, the prestyloid recess, the ulnocarpal ligaments (ulnotriquetral and ulnolunate) and the volar and dorsal distal radioulnar ligaments. Evaluate for fraying, synovitis, or loose bodies.

- Mid-carpal evaluation *(Fig. 7-8)*
  - Create the MC-R portal 1 cm distal to the 3-4 portal. Introduce the arthroscope in the usual fashion. Care should be taken not to force the arthroscope into the joint because significant chondral damage can occur.

  - The MC-U portal is established under direct visualization and a probe is placed into the mid-carpal joint.

  - Orient the visual field so that the proximal carpal row is on the bottom of the screen; the distal row on the top.

  - Capitohamate joint
    ▸ First identify the capitohamate joint by looking ulnarly. The capitohamate joint will have the appearance of a "baby's bottom" *(Fig. 7.8)*.

    ▸ The triquetrum is identified proximally, just past the capitohamate joint.

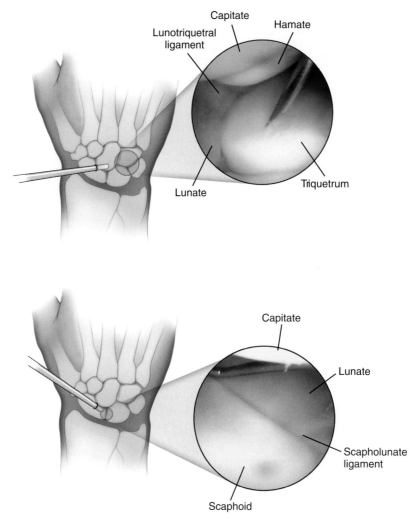

Figure 7-8. Diagnostic arthroscopy of the midcarpal joint. *(From Chhabra AB. Wrist and hand. In Miller MD, Chhabra AB, Hurwitz S, et al. [eds]. Orthopaedic Surgical Approaches. Philadelphia, Elsevier, 2008; p 193.)*

- Scaphoid-trapezium-trapezoid (STT) joint
  - ▶ Looking radially, slide the scope dorsally and radially up the scaphoid to examine the STT joint.
  - ■ Scapholunate ligament
    - ▶ The arthroscope is then brought back to a neutral position and oriented downward to view the SLL.
    - ▶ The probe is then inserted into the MC-U portal and its tip placed between the scaphoid and the lunate at the SLL to evaluate for an SLL tear. Attempt to drive the probe into the

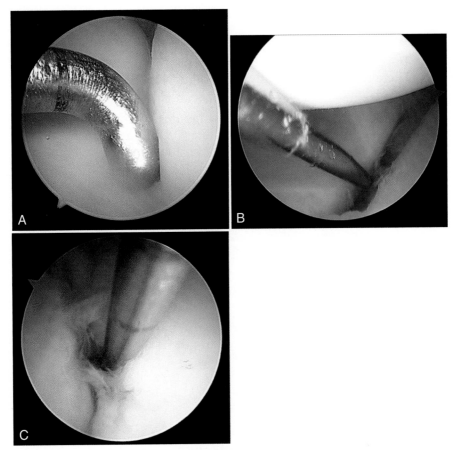

Figure 7-9. Geissler classification of SLL tears: **A**. Grade I—Probe unable to penetrate SL interval. **B**. Grade II—Probe able to penetrate interval. **C**. Grade III—Probe able to penetrate interval and rotate.

SL interval *(Fig. 7-9)*; the Giessler classification of SLL tears is outlined in *Table 7-1*.

Table 7-1. Giessler Classification of SLL Tears

Grade 1	Attenuation and/or hemorrhage of the SLL viewed from the radiocarpal joint; NO laxity noted from midcarpal joint, probe not able to penetrate the SL interval.
Grade 2	Probe can be placed into the SL interval indicating diastasis (note: this may be physiologically normal in a ligamentously lax individual).
Grade 3	Probe can be placed into the SL interval AND rotated.
Grade 4	2.7-mm arthroscope can be placed into the SL interval.

SL, scapholunate ligament; SLL, suspected scapholunate ligament.

- Lunotriquetral ligament

  ▸ Looking ulnarly and down, the lunate and LTL can be identified.

  ▸ The probe is placed into the LT interval to evaluate for laxity. There is often significantly more motion at the LT joint than the SL joint.

  ▸ Examine the lunate facet. Type 1 lunates have a singular facet for articulation of the capitate; Type 2 lunates have a double facet and also articulate with the hamate. Patients with type 2 lunates have a higher incidence of proximal pole hamate arthritis which is evident as chondromalacia during arthroscopic examination *(Fig. 7-10)*.

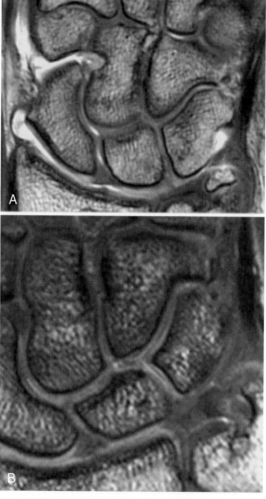

Figure 7-10. MR images: **A.** Type I lunate. **B.** Type II lunate. *(From Gill LE, Chhabra B. The role of arthroscopic evaluation and débridement in wrist arthritis. In Chhabra AB, Isaaca JE [eds]. Arthritis and Arthroplasty: The Hand, Wrist and Elbow. Philadelphia, Elsevier, 2009; p 20.)*

- Distal radioulnar joint evaluation

  - Establish the DRUJ viewing portal in the usual fashion.

  - Looking distally and radially, examine the radial and ulnar portions of the DRUJ and the proximal surface of the TFCC.

Common Arthroscopic Procedures

Débridement and Synovectomy, Removal of Loose Bodies (Debridement CPT 29846, Synovectomy Partial/Complete CPT 29844/29845)*(Fig. 7-11)*

- Débridement and synovectomy are performed in much the same manner as a diagnostic arthroscopy. The procedure begins in the radiocarpal joint through the 3-4 and 4-5 portals. A shaver or grasper is placed into the joint for removal of synovitis, debris, and loose bodies. It is important to have good outflow for a clear visual field. The portals can be interchanged to maximize access to the joint. The midcarpal joint should also be examined and débrided as necessary.

- **TFCC débridement and repair (CPT 29846)** *(Fig. 7-12)* TFCC tears have been classified by Palmer into traumatic (class I) and degenerative (class II) lesions *(Table 7-2)*. Degenerative lesions (Class IIA-E) usually involve the central portion of the TFC and usually require débridement only. If ulnar positive variance is present, a wafer procedure or ulnar shortening osteotomy should be considered. Traumatic lesions (class IA-D) may be

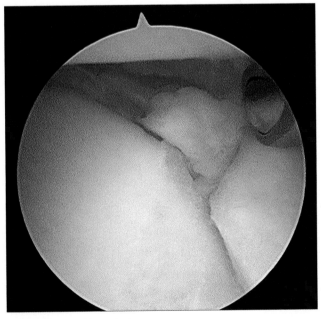

Figure 7-11. Arthroscopic view of loose body.

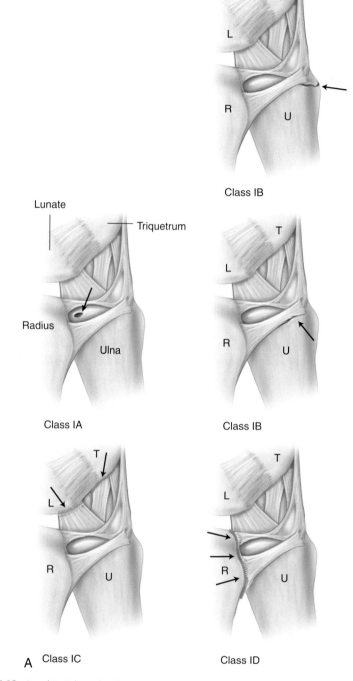

Figure 7-12. **A** and **B.** Palmer classification of TFCC tears. Class I traumatic; Class II degenerative. See Table 7-2. Arrows indicate location of tear. *(From Palmer AK. Triangular fibrocartilage complex lesions: a classification. J Hand Surg [Am] 14:594, 1989.)*

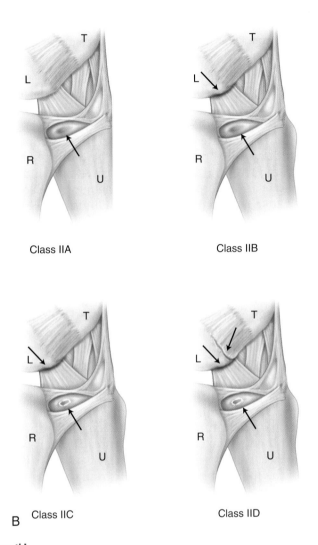

Class IIA

Class IIB

B   Class IIC

Class IID

Figure 7-12—cont'd.

Table 7-2. Palmer Classification of TFCC Tears

Traumatic Class I Tears	Degenerative Class II tears
IA: Central TFC perforation	IIA: Thinning of cartilage disc
IB: Base of ulnar styloid with or without styloid fracture	IIB: Thinning of disc and lunate chondromalacia
IC: Carpal detachment (volar ulnolunate ligaments)	IIC: Central TFC perforation and lunate chondromalacia
ID: Radial detachment with or without radial avulsion fracture	IID: Central TFC perforation, lunate chondromalacia, LTL tear
	IIE: As above, plus ulnocarpal arthritis

TFCC, triangular fibrocartilage complex.

treated with débridement or repair because the periphery of the TFC has adequate blood supply for healing. Class IA tears (central TFC perforations) generally require only débridement. Class IB tears require repair and several techniques have been described.

- In general, all TFCC débridement and repairs begin the same: Establish the 3-4 and 4-5 portals for a thorough evaluation of the radiocarpal joint. Débride extraneous tissue to have a clear view of the TFC and evaluate for tears. Perform the trampoline test on the TFC with a probe in the 4-5 portal. Note the location and severity of the tear and if there is any corresponding lunate chondromalacia. Perform gentle débridement to clean the flap edges and take care to avoid over-débriding. The 6R or 6U portal may be used as an adjunct working portal.

- For class IB tears at the base of the ulnar styloid, one of three repair techniques may be used.

- **Whipple outside-in technique** *(Fig. 7-13)*. The 3-4 portal is used as the viewing portal and the 6R portal is established under visualization for working. First a 12- to 15-mm longitudinal incision is made along the plane of and incorporating the 6R portal. The ECU tendon retinaculum is opened and the tendon is retracted volarly or dorsally. A curved cannulated needle is inserted under and through the TFC on the far side of the tear. A wire loop is placed through a cannula in the 6R portal. 2-0 PDS suture is passed through the curved needle into the joint under visualization and captured by the wire loop from the 6R portal. The loop is then retracted with the suture. This is repeated 3 or 4 times as necessary to repair the tear. All suture is then tied outside of the joint capsule—the ECU is replaced, its retinaculum is repaired, and the skin in closed.

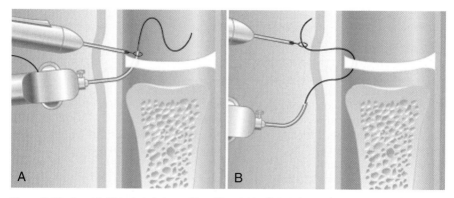

Figure 7-13. **A** and **B.** Whipple technique. *(From Chow J, Katolik L. Arthroscopic management of triangular fibrocartilage complex tears. In Miller MD, Cole BJ [eds]. Textbook of Arthroscopy. Philadelphia, Elsevier, 2004; p 420.)*

■ **Poehling inside-out technique** *(Fig. 7-14).* The 4-5 portal is used for viewing and a 20-gauge Touhy needle enters the radiocarpal joint through either the 1-2 or 3-4 portal. The needle is driven through the TFCC, capturing the tear, and out through the ligamentous tissue and skin at the ulnar aspect of the wrist. A 2-0 absorbable suture is passed through the needle and secured with a clamp on the ulnar side of the wrist. The Touhy needle is withdrawn back into the radiocarpal joint and passed again through the TFC a few millimeters from the previous stitch. Again the needle exits through the ulnar side of the wrist. This can be repeated as needed until the repair is complete. The Touhy needle is removed and a small incision is made near the suture ends. Blunt dissection is carried down to the joint capsule and the sutures are tied over the capsule and the skin is closed. Care should be taken to protect the dorsal ulnar cutaneous nerve

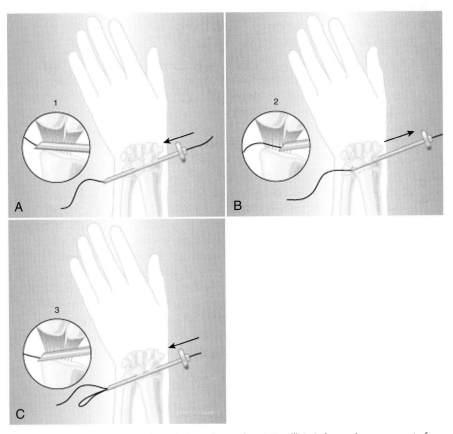

Figure 7-14. A through C. Poehling technique. *(From Chow J, Katolik L. Arthroscopic management of triangular fibrocartilage complex tears. In Miller MD, Cole BJ [eds]. Textbook of Arthroscopy. Philadelphia, Elsevier, 2004; p 421.)*

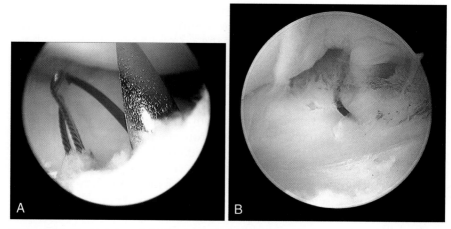

Figure 7-15. Chow technique. **A.** Passing the suture through the loop. **B.** Tying the loop; repair of the tear.

branches during closure. Visualization from the 4-5 portal confirms TFC repair during suture tying. Alternatively, the sutures can be tied over a bolster.

■ **Chow technique** *(Fig. 7-15)*. This technique is similar to the Whipple technique in principle but utilizes a meniscus suture set. The 3-4 portal is used for viewing and the 4-5 and 6R are used for working. A 25-gauge needle is first introduced into the TFCC, capturing the tear under direct visualization. This needle acts only as a guide for the straight needles. Next, a straight needle containing a wire loop is introduced through the TFC in the same plane as the guide needle. A few millimeters inferior to this first straight needle, a second straight needle containing a 2-0 suture is passed into the TFC. A grasper is placed into the 6U portal to help guide the suture through the wire loop. The straight needle holding the suture is then gently removed from the joint while the grasper secures the suture within the loop. The second straight needle is then removed to avoid cutting the suture, leaving the wire loop and suture within the joint. The loop with the captured suture is then retracted and brought out through the skin. The process may be repeated until a secure repair is achieved. A small incision is made between the suture ends to the level of the joint capsule. A probe slides under the subcutaneous tissues to bring the suture ends through the incision. The ends are tied over the capsule and the skin is closed.

Arthroscopic Ganglionectomy (CPT 29846) *(Fig. 7-16)*

- This procedure is indicated for dorsal ganglion cysts or volar ganglion cysts that are known to originate from the radiocarpal joint. The procedure begins by establishing the 4-5 portal for placement of the arthroscope. The ganglion

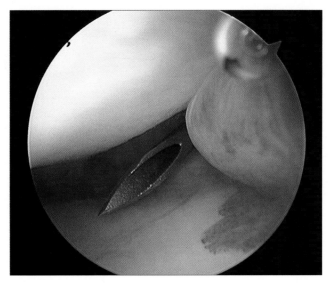

Figure 7-16. Arthroscopic view of dorsal ganglion cyst.

is identified (usually from the SLL in the case of dorsal ganglions) and the SLL is examined for instability. A needle is placed through the 3-4 portal and the ganglion is punctured. The needle is then removed and a shaver is introduced in its place. The ganglion's pedicle is identified and the entire structure is excised using the shaver until the dorsal capsule is débrided and the extensor tendons are identified. Care should be taken to avoid injury to the extensor tendons and to avoid over-débridement. It is thought that arthroscopic ganglionectomy has a lower recurrence rate than an open procedure, results in less scar formation, and provides better visualization of the origin of the ganglion. Intra-articular pathology is identified and can be addressed as well.

Distal Radius Fracture Reduction (CPT 29847) *(Fig. 7-17)*

• Intra-articular step-offs of >1 to 2 mm after distal radius fracture can result in traumatic arthritis of the radiocarpal joint. Arthroscopic assistance may be used during reduction to help minimize this risk. Standard 3-4 and 4-5 portals are established as well as outflow on the ulnar side of the joint. First the joint is débrided of extraneous material and clot and a diagnostic arthroscopy is performed. The distal radius fracture or fractures are identified and reduction is performed using traction, Kirschner wires, and elevators as necessary. Separate skin incisions may need to be made to aid in reduction. When the joint surface has been restored and confirmed with fluoroscopy, the reduction is held in place with K-wires, screws, or plates as appropriate. More proximal portions of the fracture should be addressed only after the joint congruity has been restored.

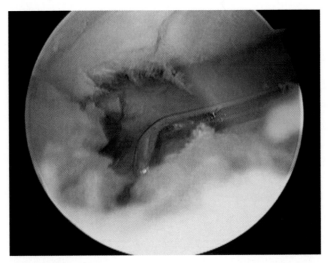

Figure 7-17. Arthroscopic view of distal radius fracture reduction.

Scaphoid Fracture Reduction (CPT 29847)
- The MC-U portal is used for viewing and the MC-R may be used for instrumentation. The midcarpal joint is débrided and the scaphoid fracture is identified. The fracture is manipulated into reduction and secured with .035 or .045 K wires. Alternatively, percutaneous compression screws may also be used. Arthroscopy is very helpful to ensure that the articular surfaces of the scaphoid and lunate are not violated.

Scapholunate Ligament Repair (CPT 29847) *(Fig. 7-18 SLL and LTL repair)*
- A diagnostic arthroscopy is performed to grade the SLL injury. Grade I tears require only ligament débridement from the radiocarpal portals. Reducible grade 2 or 3 tears require débridement and fixation. The 3-4 portal is used for viewing and the 4-5 portal is used for instrumentation. The SLL is identified and débrided with a shaver. One .045 K wire is driven into the dorsal aspect of the lunate and one into the scaphoid to act as joysticks. To correct the deformity, the scaphoid is extended and the lunate is flexed. Once reduced under arthroscopic visualization and confirmed on fluoroscopy, two K wires are driven from the scaphoid into the lunate and at least one K wire is driven from the scaphoid into the capitate.

Lunotriquetral Ligament Repair (CPT 29847) *(see Fig. 7-18 SLL and LTL repair)*
- LTL injuries rarely occur as an isolated injury and arthroscopic repair can be technically demanding. The procedure begins with a diagnostic arthroscopy to evaluate for concomitant injuries. If the LTL is partially torn, débridement is sufficient. If the tear is complete, repair is necessary to correct the

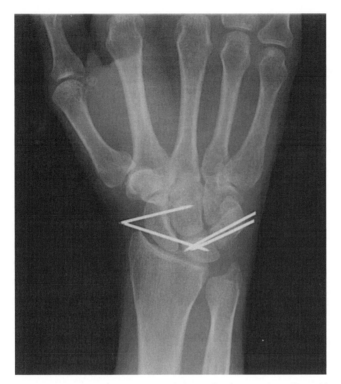

Figure 7-18. Lunotriquetral ligament repair and scapholunate ligament repair. Radiographic postreduction and repair.

resulting deformity. The 3-4 portal is used for viewing and an 18-gauge needle is passed into the 6U portal under visualization. The ulnolunate and ulnotriquetral ligaments are identified and a straight needle with a wire loop is passed through the 6R portal. A 2-0 PDS suture is passed into the 18-gauge needle, capturing the UL and UT ligaments, and is passed into the wire loop to be brought out the 6R portal. Pressure is applied to the lunate and tension is placed on the suture surrounding the UL and UT ligaments. This maneuver should reduce the VISI deformity. Two .045 K wires are driven from the triquetrum to the lunate and at least one K wire is driven from the triquetrum to the hamate. Fluoroscopy confirms that the deformity is corrected. The traction tower is released and the suture is tied subcutaneously.

Kienböck's Disease Grading (CPT 29840) *(Fig. 7-19)*

● A diagnostic arthroscopy for grading of Kienböck's disease can help determine the correct treatment modality such as joint leveling procedure, proximal row carpectomy, or wrist arthrodesis. The lunate and its articulating surfaces are evaluated during a diagnostic arthroscopy from both the radiocarpal and midcarpal joints. *Table 7-3* describes the grading system.

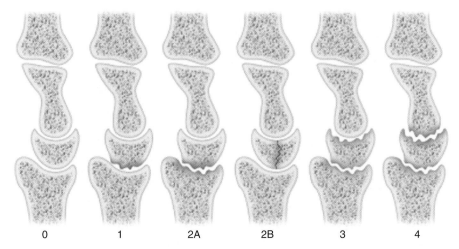

| 0 | 1 | 2A | 2B | 3 | 4 |

Figure 7-19. Arthroscopic staging of Kienböck's disease. Grade 0. Identified on MRI but no evidence of cartilage loss; synovitis may be present. Grade 1. Chondral defects on proximal lunate. Grade 2A. Chondral defects on lunate facet of radius. Grade 2B. Chondral defects with coronal lunate fracture. Grade 3. Chondral defects proximal and distal lunate and lunate facet of radius. Grade 4. Chondral defects proximal and distal lunate, lunate facet of radius, and proximal capitate. See also Table 7-3. *(From Gill LE, Chhabra AB. The role of arthroscopic evaluation and débridement in wrist arthritis. In Chhabra AB, Isaacs JE [eds]. Arthritis and Arthroplasty: The Hand, Wrist and Elbow. Philadelphia, Elsevier, 2010; p 18.)*

Table 7-3. Arthroscopic Grading of Kienböck's Disease

Grade	Description	Treatment
0	Identified on MRI but no evidence of cartilage loss; synovitis may be present	Débridement and/or joint leveling procedure
1	Chondral defects on proximal lunate	Proximal row carpectomy, limited wrist arthrodesis, lunate excision, and scaphocapitate arthrodesis
2	(A) Chondral defects on lunate facet of radius; (B) Chondral defects with coronal lunate fracture	Proximal row carpectomy or limited wrist arthrodesis
3	Chondral defects proximal and distal lunate and lunate facet of radius	Total wrist arthrodesis or arthroplasty
4	Chondral defects proximal and distal lunate, lunate facet of radius, and proximal capitate	Total wrist arthrodesis or arthroplasty

Proximal Pole Hamate Débridement (CPT 29846)

- Arthritis of the proximal pole of the hamate can occur in patients with type II lunates because of the lunate articulation with the hamate and can cause ulnar-sided wrist pain. Arthroscopic examination of the proximal pole of the hamate allows for evaluation of the articular cartilage and for concomitant injuries to the LTL or TFCC. Treatment can consist of arthroscopic chondroplasty or proximal pole excision. To perform an excision, the arthroscope is placed in the MC-R portal and a 2.9-mm burr is placed into the MC-U portal. Approximately one burr's diameter (average 2.4 mm) of the proximal pole of the hamate should be excised. The arthroscope and burr portals can be switched for better visualization and access. Excision of the proximal pole of the hamate has proved to be a very effective treatment method, especially if the arthritis occurs as an isolated entity. Good results are also reported with proximal pole hamate excision and LTL injury.

Ulnar Wafer Resection/Ulnar Shortening (CPT 29846) *(Fig. 7-20)*

- This is an alternative to an open procedure. First a diagnostic arthroscopy is performed to evaluate for LTL instability, degenerative tears of the TFCC, and chondromalacia of the lunate or ulnar head. The 3-4 portal is used for viewing and the 6U or 6R portal is used for instrumentation. The ulnar side of the radiocarpal joint is débrided for visualization. The TFCC is identified and the central portion of the articular disc is débrided circumferentially until only the peripheral one third remains, thereby revealing the underlying ulnar head.

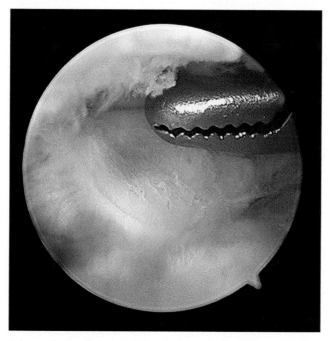

Figure 7-20. Arthroscopic view of ulnar shortening—exposing the distal ulna.

The distal DRUJ portal is established with a needle under direct visualization from the 3-4 portal. The level of the needle should be just below the remaining fibrocartilage and just above the ulnar head at the level of the sigmoid notch. A burr is placed into the 6R or 6U portal and the ulnar head is meticulously shaved to the level of the burr (2.9 mm). The forearm is rotated to allow complete resection of the ulnar head through the hole in the fibrocartilage. Take care to avoid over-resection by using intraoperative fluoroscopy frequently. If there are areas of the ulnar head that are difficult to reach, the burr may be placed into the distal DRUJ portal to complete the resection.

Complications

The complication rate with wrist arthroscopy is rare and thought to be around 2%. A thorough knowledge of wrist anatomy and meticulous portal placement can prevent most complications.

- Neurovascular injury
  - The superficial sensory radial nerve and the radial artery are at risk for injury during placement of the 1-2 portal.
  - The dorsal cutaneous branch of the ulnar nerve is at risk during placement of the 6U portal and during TFCC repair if a suture is tied over the nerve in the subcutaneous tissues.
  - The cutaneous branch of the median nerve can be injured during placement of the VR portal.
  - The ulnar nerve can be injured during placement of the VU portal.
  - Neurovascular injury is prevented by accurate placement of portals and by sharp instrumentation of SKIN ONLY. Blunt dissection should commence through the subcutaneous tissues and blunt trochars should be used during portal placement.

- Tendon and ligament injury
  - The most commonly injured tendon is the extensor pollicis longus (EPL) during placement of the 3-4 portal.
  - The EPL and extensor indicis are at risk of injury during placement of the 3-4 portal.
  - The extensor carpi ulnaris and extensor digiti minimi are at risk during placement of the 6R portal.
  - The common extensor tendons are at risk of injury during placement of either midcarpal portal.
  - The SLL can be injured by sharp deep instrumentation through the 3-4 portal.

- The TFCC can be injured by sharp instrumentation through the 6R or 6U portal.

- The FCR can be injured during placement of the VR portal if not properly retracted and protected.

- The FCU can be injured during placement of the VU portal if not properly retracted.

- Tendon and ligament injuries are prevented by accurate portal placement and by sharp instrumentation of the SKIN ONLY. Blunt dissection should commence through the subcutaneous tissues and blunt trochars should be used during portal placement. An instrument should NEVER be forced into a portal. High resistance most likely indicates an interposed tendon. Also, portals should be established under direct visualization to avoid intra-articular injuries.

- Chondral injury
  - Articular cartilage is at risk during the placement of the trochar, arthroscope, and various instruments through the portals.

  - Risk of injury is minimized with accurate portal placement, gentle introduction of instruments, and by not forcing any instruments into the joint.

- Traction injuries
  - Nylon finger traps should be used to minimize tearing and cutting of the skin on the fingers, especially in patients with rheumatoid arthritis or poor skin turgor.

  - Minimize the surgical time under traction so as to avoid traction injuries to peripheral nerves; do not place more than 15 lb of traction across the wrist.

- Loss of ROM
  - Some transient mild loss of ROM is expected from post-operative swelling and immobilization.

  - Minimize scar tissue by meticulous portal placement.

  - Occupational therapy should be used judiciously in the post-operative period for edema control and ROM exercises. Pain control should be adequate to facilitate movement.

- Compartment syndrome
  - Can occur during arthroscopically assisted distal radius fracture reduction. Lower the risk by the use of gravity inflow, working efficiently to minimize surgery duration, frequent monitoring of the forearm for edema, and by delaying surgery until at least 3 days from the date of injury.

- Infection
  - Superficial infections can occur but risk is reduced by administration of preoperative antibiotics.
  - If K wires are used, it is suggested that the wires are cut and buried beneath the skin to lower the chance for a pin tract infection which could lead to a septic joint or osteomyelitis.

REFERENCES

Bain GI, Munt J, and Turner PC. New advances in wrist arthroscopy. *Arthroscopy: J Arthrop Rel Surg* 2008; 24(3):355–367.

Beredihiklian PK, Bozentka DJ, Leung YL, and Monaghan BA. *Complications of wrist arthroscopy. J Hand Surg* 2004; 29A(3):406–411.

Chhabra AB. Wrist and hand. In Miller MD, Chhabra AB, and Hurwitz S, et al. (eds). *Orthopaedic Surgical Approaches*, Philadelphia, Elsevier, 2008; pp 145–210.

Chloros GD, Wiesler ER, and Poehling GG. Current concepts in wrist arthro-scopy. *Arthroscopy* 2008; 24(3):343–354.

Culp RW. Complications of wrist arthroscopy. In Culp RW (ed). *Wrist and Hand Arthroscopy. Hand Clinics,* Philadelphia, Saunders, 1999; 15(3), pp 529–535.

de Araujo W, Poehling GG, and Kuzma GR. New Tuohy needle technique for triangular fibrocartilage complex repair: preliminary studies *Arthroscopy: J Arthrop Rel Surg* 1996; 12(6):699–703.

Hornbach EE and Osterman AL. Partial excision of the triangular fibrocartilage complex. In Gleberman RH (ed). *The Wrist*, Philadelphia, Lippincott Williams & Wilkins, 2002; pp 279–290.

Katolik LI and Fernandez JJ. Arthroscopy of the wrist and hand. In Miller MD and Chhabra BJ (eds). *Textbook of Arthroscopy*, Philadelphia, Elsevier, 2004; pp 371–426.

Poehling GG and Williams RMM. Arthroscopic repair of the triangular fibro-cartilage complex. In Gleberman RH (ed). *The Wrist*, Philadelphia, Lippincott Williams & Wilkins, 2002; pp 291–306.

Savoie FH III and Field LD. Diagnostic and operative arthroscopy. In Gleberman RH (ed). *The Wrist*, Philadelphia, Lippincott Williams & Wilkins, 2002; pp 19–35.

Slutsky DJ and Nagle DJ. Wrist arthroscopy: current concepts. *J Hand Surg* 2008; 33A:1228–1244.

INDEX

Note: Page numbers followed by *f* indicate figures and *t* indicate tables.

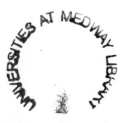